REPORT DOCUMENTATION PAGE

Form Approved
OMB No. 0704-0188

Public reporting burden for this collection of information is estimated to average 1 hour per response, including the time for reviewing instructions, searching existing data sources, gathering and maintaining the data needed, and completing and reviewing the collection of information. Send comments regarding this burden estimate or any other aspect of this collection of information, including suggestions for reducing this burden, to Washington Headquarters Services, Directorate for Information Operations and Reports, 1215 Jefferson Davis Highway, Suite 1204, Arlington, VA 22202-4302, and to the Office of Management and Budget, Paperwork Reduction Project (0704-0188), Washington, DC 20503.

1. AGENCY USE ONLY (Leave blank)	2. REPORT DATE March 2002	3. REPORT TYPE AND DATES COVERED Final Report March 2002

4. TITLE AND SUBTITLE
Best Practices Manual: FTA Drug and Alcohol Testing Program

5. FUNDING NUMBERS
U2027/TM254

6. AUTHOR(S)
Robert L. Gaumer

7. PERFORMING ORGANIZATION NAME(S) AND ADDRESS(ES)
EG&G Technical Services *
55 Broadway
Cambridge, MA 02142-1093

8. PERFORMING ORGANIZATION REPORT NUMBER
DOT-VNTSC-FTA-02-05

9. SPONSORING/MONITORING AGENCY NAME(S) AND ADDRESS(ES)
U.S. Department of Transportation
Federal Transit Administration
Office of Safety and Security
Washington, DC 20590

10. SPONSORING/MONITORING AGENCY REPORT NUMBER
FTA-MA-90-5005-02-1

11. SUPPLEMENTARY NOTES
*Under contract to:
U.S. Department of Transportation
Research and Special Programs Administration
John A. Volpe National Transportation Systems Center
55 Broadway
Cambridge, MA 02142-0193

12a. DISTRIBUTION/AVAILABILITY STATEMENT
This document is available to the public through the National Technical Information Service, Springfield, Virginia 22161.

12b. DISTRIBUTION CODE

13. ABSTRACT (Maximum 200 words)
This document is part of a two-volume set prepared under the Federal Transit Administration's (FTA) General Technical Assistance Program, to provide guidance to the recipients of FTA funding that are required to test their safety-sensitive employees for drug use and alcohol misuse. This volume discusses "best practices" used by employers to establish and maintain a compliant testing program. The other volume, *Implementation Guidelines for Drug and Alcohol Regulations in Mass Transit*, explains the regulatory requirements, which were revised in 2001.

The best practices discussed here were identified during 5 years of FTA-sponsored audits of existing programs. They are responses to the requirements that allow for flexibility in how to comply, i.e., areas where employers have to choose between different options and areas where they may want to exceed the minimum FTA requirements. This document identifies the areas where choices are required, the issues involved in making those choices, and "real world" examples of choices made. The discussions are organized according to the four required elements of an FTA anti-drug use and alcohol misuse program: (1) a program policy statement, (2) an education and training program, (3) a testing program, and (4) a procedure for referring policy violators to a substance abuse professional.

14. SUBJECT TERMS
Drugs and alcohol, drug and alcohol testing, best practices, public transit, safety, accidents, Federal Transit Administration, FTA, regulations.

15. NUMBER OF PAGES
328

16. PRICE CODE

17. SECURITY CLASSIFICATION OF REPORT Unclassified	18. SECURITY CLASSIFICATION OF THIS PAGE Unclassified	19. SECURITY CLASSIFICATION OF ABSTRACT Unclassified	20. LIMITATION OF ABSTRACT Unlimited

METRIC/ENGLISH CONVERSION FACTORS

ENGLISH TO METRIC

LENGTH (APPROXIMATE)

1 inch (in)	= 2.5 centimeters (cm)
1 foot (ft)	= 30 centimeters (cm)
1 yard (yd)	= 0.9 meter (m)
1 mile (mi)	= 1.6 kilometers (km)

AREA (APPROXIMATE)

1 square inch (sq in, in^2)	= 6.5 square centimeters (cm^2)
1 square foot (sq ft, ft^2)	= 0.09 square meter (m^2)
1 square yard (sq yd, yd^2)	= 0.8 square meter (m^2)
1 square mile (sq mi, mi^2)	= 2.6 square kilometers (km^2)
1 acre = 0.4 hectare (he)	= 4,000 square meters (m^2)

MASS - WEIGHT (APPROXIMATE)

1 ounce (oz)	= 28 grams (gm)
1 pound (lb)	= 0.45 kilogram (kg)
1 short ton = 2,000 pounds (lb)	= 0.9 tonne (t)

VOLUME (APPROXIMATE)

1 teaspoon (tsp)	= 5 milliliters (ml)
1 tablespoon (tbsp)	= 15 milliliters (ml)
1 fluid ounce (fl oz)	= 30 milliliters (ml)
1 cup (c)	= 0.24 liter (l)
1 pint (pt)	= 0.47 liter (l)
1 quart (qt)	= 0.96 liter (l)
1 gallon (gal)	= 3.8 liters (l)
1 cubic foot (cu ft, ft^3)	= 0.03 cubic meter (m^3)
1 cubic yard (cu yd, yd^3)	= 0.76 cubic meter (m^3)

TEMPERATURE (EXACT)

$[(x-32)(5/9)]$ °F = y °C

METRIC TO ENGLISH

LENGTH (APPROXIMATE)

1 millimeter (mm)	= 0.04 inch (in)
1 centimeter (cm)	= 0.4 inch (in)
1 meter (m)	= 3.3 feet (ft)
1 meter (m)	= 1.1 yards (yd)
1 kilometer (km)	= 0.6 mile (mi)

AREA (APPROXIMATE)

1 square centimeter (cm^2)	= 0.16 square inch (sq in, in^2)
1 square meter (m^2)	= 1.2 square yards (sq yd, yd^2)
1 square kilometer (km^2)	= 0.4 square mile (sq mi, mi^2)
10,000 square meters (m^2)	= 1 hectare (ha) = 2.5 acres

MASS - WEIGHT (APPROXIMATE)

1 gram (gm)	= 0.036 ounce (oz)
1 kilogram (kg)	= 2.2 pounds (lb)
1 tonne (t)	= 1,000 kilograms (kg)
	= 1.1 short tons

VOLUME (APPROXIMATE)

1 milliliter (ml)	= 0.03 fluid ounce (fl oz)
1 liter (l)	= 2.1 pints (pt)
1 liter (l)	= 1.06 quarts (qt)
1 liter (l)	= 0.26 gallon (gal)
1 cubic meter (m^3)	= 36 cubic feet (cu ft, ft^3)
1 cubic meter (m^3)	= 1.3 cubic yards (cu yd, yd^3)

TEMPERATURE (EXACT)

$[(9/5) y + 32]$ °C = x °F

QUICK INCH - CENTIMETER LENGTH CONVERSION

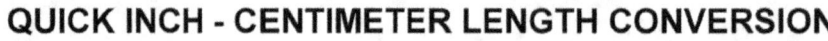
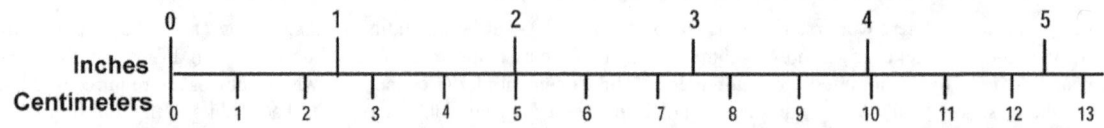

QUICK FAHRENHEIT - CELSIUS TEMPERATURE CONVERSION

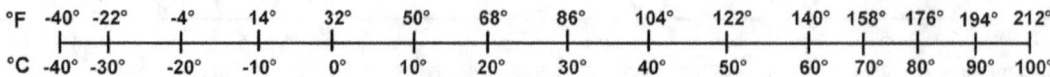

For more exact and or other conversion factors, see NIST Miscellaneous Publication 286, Units of Weights and Measures. Price $2.50 SD Catalog No. C13 10286

Updated 6/17/98

Preface

In 1995, the Federal Transit Administration (FTA) established an on-site audit program to monitor compliance with the drug and alcohol testing regulations enacted by the U.S. Department of Transportation in 49 CFR Part 40, *Procedures for Transportation Workplace Drug and Alcohol Testing Programs*, and by FTA in 49 CFR Part 653, *Prevention of Prohibited Drug Use in Transit Operations*, and 49 CFR Part 654, *Prevention of Alcohol Misuse in Transit Operations*. The many audits conducted under this program have revealed efficient and effective methods used by recipients of FTA funding to comply with the many areas of flexibility in those regulations. These methods are referred to as "best practices."

This document discusses the issues that employers should address when deciding how to comply with and whether to exceed the DOT/FTA requirements, and provides best practice examples (identified during the audits) of decisions made by the audited entities. The examples are responses to the various regulatory requirements. Also included are multiple responses to the same requirements to show different approaches used by different types of employers. Because the workforces and operating environments of FTA funding recipients vary widely in some respects, the material in every example will probably not be applicable to every entity, and in some cases none of the examples may be applicable word-for-word.

This *Best Practices* manual assumes that the reader understands the regulatory requirements, which are explained in *Implementation Guidelines for Drug and Alcohol Regulations in Mass Transit*. The *Implementation Guidelines* document updates the document published under the same title in April 1994 *(FTA-OH-26-001-94-1)*. The revised *Implementation Guidelines* summarize and interpret the revised 49 CFR Part 40 issued in December 2000 and the revised FTA regulations, issued in August 2001 in 49 CFR Part 655, *Prevention of Alcohol Misuse and Drug Use in Transit*.

All of the examples in this manual were audited and judged to be compliant with Part 40 before it was recently revised and with Parts 653 and 654. Each of the example policy statements (contained in Appendix A, and discussed and referenced in Chapter 2) have been updated to address the revised Part 40 and Part 655, but no policies have been audited for compliance with the revised Part 40 and Part 655. The other best practice examples have been adjusted by the author to reflect the revisions in Parts 40 and 655.

This manual will be posted on the FTA Office of Safety and Security website: http://transit-safety.volpe.dot.gov, and will be updated periodically. The web posting will probably be updated more often than the printed document.

Acknowledgements

The author wishes to thank Mark Snider of the Federal Transit Administration (FTA) Office of Safety and Security for his guidance and direction in preparing this manual. The author also thanks James Harrison of the Volpe National Transportation Systems Center for his direction and coordination of the various resources required for this project. Special appreciation is given to Robbie Sarles and Jeff Halstead of RLS & Associates for their invaluable assistance in providing information and best practice examples, for providing contacts for additional examples, and for reviewing the draft text and appendices. Rodney Sams of ICF Consulting and Leila Procopio-Makuh of LPM and Associates also provided information and best practice examples. John Morrison of Ketron reviewed the technical accuracy of the text and policy examples. Appreciation is given to the many transit agencies and state departments of transportation that contributed examples of their practices. These include:

- Broward County (Florida) Transit
- City of Albuquerque, Transit Department
- Denver Regional Transit District
- Des Moines Metropolitan Transportation Authority
- Government of the Virgin Islands
- Greater Cleveland Regional Transit Authority (GCRTA)
- Hartford (Connecticut) Regional Transit District
- Long Beach (California) Transit
- Los Angeles County Metropolitan Transportation Authority (LACMTA)
- Massachusetts Bay Transportation Authority (MBTA)
- Rhode Island Public Transit Authority (RIPTA)
- San Francisco Bay Area Rapid Transit (BART) District
- Southeastern Pennsylvania Transportation Authority (SEPTA)
- Southwestern Ohio Regional Transit Authority (SORTA)/Cincinnati Metro
- SuTran Transit System, Sioux Falls, South Dakota
- Tri-County Metropolitan Transit District, Oregon/Tri-Met
- Washington Metropolitan Area Transportation Authority (WMATA)
- Western Maine Transportation Services
- Florida Department of Transportation
- Georgia Department of Transportation
- Minnesota Department of Transportation
- Ohio Department of Transportation
- West Virginia Department of Transportation, Division of Public Transit

The author also thanks Nathan Grace of EG&G Technical Services for assisting with the review process and coordinating the production of this manual.

Table of Contents

List of Figures

1. Introduction

This *Best Practices* manual discusses issues in the US Department of Transportation's (US DOT) and Federal Transit Administration's (FTA) drug and alcohol testing regulations where employers have to make decisions on how to comply with the requirements, and provides "real world" examples of choices made. This manual and *Implementation Guidelines for Drug and Alcohol Regulations in Mass Transit* are being issued as a two-volume set under the FTA's General Technical Assistance Program, to provide guidance to the FTA grantees that are required to test their safety-sensitive employees for drug use and alcohol misuse. The *Best Practices* manual assumes that the reader understands the regulatory requirements, which are explained in the *Implementation Guidelines*.

1.1 Background

In 1991, in response to growing concerns about the risks posed by the use of drugs and misuse of alcohol by transportation industry employees while performing safety-sensitive functions, Congress passed *The Omnibus Transportation Employee Testing Act*, which mandated all agencies of US DOT to implement a drug and alcohol testing program. In 1994, US DOT published the minimum uniform requirements for the programs of all the modal administrations, in 49 CFR Part 40, *Procedures for Transportation Workplace Drug and Alcohol Testing Programs*.

Also in 1994, FTA published requirements for certain recipients of FTA financial assistance, in 49 CFR Part 653, *Prevention of Prohibited Drug Use in Transit Operations*, and 49 CFR Part 654, *Prevention of Alcohol Misuse in Transit Operations*. The FTA regulations were consistent with the provisions of Part 40. They were designed to provide the maximum level of safety to passengers using public transit services across the country, the employees of such providers, and others who may share the roadway with transit vehicles; to protect civil rights; and to minimize liability in all locations.

Shortly after the FTA regulations were implemented, FTA initiated a program to monitor compliance. Monitoring consists of review of annual reports submitted by the grantees, as required by the regulations, and on-site audits of the grantees' drug and alcohol testing programs. The number of transit accidents per passenger mile involving operators, dispatchers, and others who control the movement of vehicles has decreased since the program was initiated.

In 2000, US DOT revised Part 40, to clarify the organization and language, to incorporate guidance and interpretations, and to respond to changes in technology and the testing industry. The amended Part 40 was published in the *Federal Register* in December 2000.

Accordingly, the FTA regulations were revised to conform with the amended Part 40. The revised FTA drug and alcohol regulations were combined in a single rule: 49 CFR Part 655, *Prevention of Alcohol Misuse and Drug Use in Transit.* The revised rule also incorporates comments from the FTA grantees and guidance that FTA has issued in the past several years, including technical assistance, letters of interpretation, audit findings, newsletters, training classes, safety seminars, and public speaking engagements.

1.2 Scope of Best Practices

Although some of the FTA testing requirements are rigid and prescriptive with straight forward responses, many of the requirements have no single response that would be correct for all grantees. There are areas of flexibility requiring decisions on how to comply. Part 655 also allows employers to exceed its minimum requirements.

This document discusses the issues that employers should factor into their decisions of how to comply with and whether to exceed the FTA requirements. It also provides the numerous "best practices" identified during the many on-site audits conducted over the past several years. "Best Practices" are efficient and effective methods used by grantees to comply with the requirements.

The practices in this document include policy statements, forms and checklists, and narrative descriptions of approaches actually used by grantees. In some cases, multiple examples for addressing the same issue or requirement are given to show different solutions for different types of transit systems or operating scenarios, or just to offer the grantees choices for achieving the same result. Though the audit teams have found the grantees to be very similar in general, they have found them to be very different in specifics. Therefore, the material in every example will probably not be applicable to every entity, and in some cases none of the examples may be applicable word-for-word.

The companion to this document, *Implementation Guidelines for Drug and Alcohol Regulations in Mass Transit,* updates the document published under the same title in April 1994 (FTA-OH-26-001-94-1). The revised *Implementation Guidelines* summarize and interpret Part 655. The *Implementation Guidelines* and the *Best Practices* are intended to be used together; each document provides numerous cross-references to the other document. The *Implementation Guidelines* tell the reader what the requirements are, and the *Best Practices* tell how to comply with them.

1.3 Organization of Best Practices Information

This manual is designed for easy reference for specific issues or requirements, and it refers readers to the *Implementation Guidelines* for explanation of the requirements.

> The many best practice examples in this manual appear in six appendices, and are referenced and discussed in the text. The text is bound separately so it can be removed from the binder for ease of use when referring to the examples. The separately bound text can also be readily carried or stored in a pocket or briefcase for use as a portable reference.

Chapters 2 through 5 address the four required elements of a drug and alcohol testing program specified in Part 655.12. Chapter 2 addresses the program policy statement requirements and cites examples from compliant[1] policies; it is subdivided according to the many content areas specified in Part 655.15. Chapter 3 describes the types of education and training programs that have been implemented to satisfy the requirements in Part 655.14, and summarizes lengthy full-text examples that will be provided on the FTA Office of Safety and Security website: http://transit-safety.volpe.dot.gov. Chapter 4 provides best practice discussions and cites many examples for implementing and managing a drug and alcohol testing program; it is subdivided by program functions-- internal administration (the employer's own program), external administration (the program of the employer's contractors, subrecipients, and service agents), specimen collection and analysis, medical review, and records management. Chapter 5 addresses referral, treatment, and evaluation of employees who produce positive drug or alcohol test results, including procuring and monitoring substance abuse professionals (SAPs).

Appendix A contains the full-text example policies discussed in Chapter 2. Appendix B contains the example administrative forms and lists discussed in Section 4.1. Appendix C contains the example oversight forms and lists discussed in Section 4.2. Appendix D contains the example specimen collection forms and lists discussed in Section 4.3. Appendix E contains the example medical review forms and lists discussed in Section 4.4. Appendix F contains the example substance abuse referral forms discussed in Chapter 5.

> This manual will be posted on the FTA Office of Safety and Security website: http://transit-safety.volpe.dot.gov, and will be updated periodically. The web posting will probably be updated more often than the printed document.

---

[1] Each of the example policies cited in Chapter 2 (and presented in Appendix A) was audited and judged to be compliant with Part 40 before it was recently revised and with Parts 653 and 654, and each of them has been updated to address the revised Part 40 and Part 655. However, no policies have been audited for compliance with the revised Part 40 and Part 655.

2. Program Policy Statement

As mentioned in the *Implementation Guidelines* (in Chapter 4), FTA requires each employer to establish a policy that defines its Drug and Alcohol Testing Program, and requires the entity's governing body to formally adopt the policy. An entity's governing body is the board of directors or highest ranking officials. The person who is primarily responsible for implementing and managing the program usually guides development of the initial draft of the policy, and presents it to the governing body for review and approval. It is generally useful to involve top management officials, union officials (if the employees are represented), and local legal counsel in reviews of the draft policy.

To show proof of governing board adoption, some entities include a header on their entire document that contains the policy number, adoption date, and appropriate signature. Other common methods include a page documenting meeting minutes, or a formal adoption page complete with signatures. Another method is to include it as an appendix.

Although policies must be changed, readopted, and redistributed to reflect significant regulatory revisions, policy readoption is not necessary for minor regulatory changes or minor changes in the policy statement, such as the name of the entity's new Drug and Alcohol Program Manager, Medical Review Officer (MRO), Substance Abuse Professional (SAP), collection site, or testing laboratory. Such changes are often included in an appendix and described in a form distributed to safety-sensitive employees. Moreover, these types of changes can often be avoided by adding the words "or successor" after the names of specific persons and organizations.

Some employers use their own staff to develop the policy. Others contract with an outside expert or company. Both approaches have been successful. Peer systems can share their policies, but they should read the shared language carefully to make sure it meets the specific needs of their system. The key to a successful policy is that it be clear to the employees and clear to the attorneys and auditors. Clearly stated policies that focus on specifics tend to have the fewest legal challenges.

Use of a consultant may be preferable if the entity lacks the appropriate internal resources and if consultants are available who are extremely familiar with the FTA regulations and fully understand the local situation. The experience of prospective consultants should be examined carefully before they are hired. The audit teams have found a broad range in the quality of policies developed by consultants. Even some of the large consulting companies providing transportation safety support do not seem to be fully aware of the

FTA regulations. Some of them assume that Federal Motor Carrier Safety Administration (FMCSA) testing requirements are the same as those for FTA.

Appendix A contains six example policies for entities that wish to develop their policy internally or oversee the work of consultants:

(1) Southwestern Ohio Regional Transit Authority/Cincinnati Metro

(2) Long Beach Transit (California)

(3) Tri-County Metropolitan Transit District/Tri-Met (Portland, Oregon)

(4) Des Moines Metropolitan Transit Authority (Iowa)

(5) Ohio Department of Transportation

(6) Georgia Department of Transportation

Each of these policies was audited and judged to be compliant with Part 40 before it was recently revised and with Parts 653 and 654, and each of them has been updated to address the revised Part 40 and Part 655. However, no policies have been audited for compliance with the revised Part 40 and Part 655.

*The Cincinnati Metro and Long Beach Transit Policies in Appendix A have **not** been formally approved by their governing boards since they were revised.*

These six policies were chosen to provide a broad cross section of different types of grantees. Cincinnati Metro and Long Beach Transit are large bus systems. Tri-Met is a large bus and light rail system. The Des Moines Metropolitan Transit Authority (MTA) is a medium-size bus system. The Ohio Department of Transportation (DOT) and Georgia DOT each issue a model policy to all their subrecipients (almost all of which are small transit operators and most of them rural), and strongly encourage its use.

The Cincinnati Metro and Long Beach Transit Policies are zero tolerance for testing positive. The Ohio DOT Policy permits the subrecipient to specify zero tolerance or a second chance. The Des Moines MTA Policy is zero tolerance for testing positive on all tests except random, but it specifies a second chance for a random positive. The Tri-Met and Georgia DOT Policies permit a second chance but do not guarantee it.

The Long Beach Transit Policy is configured differently than the others. It is packaged as a booklet that employers and supervisors can readily carry with them. It begins with a 22-point summary of the policy, divided into three areas: illegal drug policy, FTA drug policy, and alcohol policy. The summary is followed by "guidelines" for administering the policy.

Point-by-point discussions of the minimum policy-content requirements in Part 655.15 with specific references to the examples in Appendix A are provided in the remainder of this chapter. These discussions are organized in subsections that generally correspond with the requirements, though the order has been changed to reflect the needs and preferences of the grantees and employers:

(1) **FTA Test Requirement** - The requirement that safety-sensitive employees must submit to drug and alcohol testing administered in accordance with Part 655

(2) **Optional Provisions** - Employer-implemented requirements of the drug and alcohol program that exceed the minimum requirements in Parts 40 and 655

(3) **Applicability** - The categories of employees subject to the regulations

(4) **Prohibited Behavior** – Specific information concerning the conduct that is prohibited by Part 655

(5) **Testing Circumstances** - The specific circumstances under which safety-sensitive employees will be tested for alcohol and prohibited drugs

(6) **Drug and Alcohol Testing Methodology and Integrity** - The procedures used to test for the presence of drugs and alcohol, to protect the employee and the integrity of the testing process, to safeguard the validity of the test results, and to ensure that the test results are attributed to the correct employee (A statement that the employer will follow all the requirements in 49 CFR Part 40 will suffice.)

(7) **Refusal Behavior and Consequences** - A description of the behavior that constitutes a refusal to take a drug or alcohol test and a statement that refusal constitutes a violation of the employer's policy

(8) **Consequences of a Drug or Alcohol Positive** - The consequences for an employee who has a verified positive drug test, has a verified alcohol concentration of 0.04 or greater, or refuses to submit to a drug or alcohol test (including mandatory requirements of immediate removal from the safety-sensitive function and evaluation by a SAP), and the consequences (as set forth in Part 655.35) for an employee who has a verified alcohol concentration of 0.02 or greater but less than 0.04

(9) **Designated Contact Person** - The identity of the person designated by the employer to answer employee questions about the drug and alcohol program

Many policies combine these categories and include additional categories. Training and education often appear in policy statements, though not required by Part 655.15. The Tri-Met Policy (in Section L), the Ohio DOT Policy (in Section D), and the Long Beach Transit Guidelines (in Section V) include a section on education and training. The Cincinnati Metro Policy (in Part III Section 9.0) and the Georgia DOT Policy (in Section 9.0) include a section on training.

2.1 FTA Test Requirement

A statement that covered employees must submit to drug and alcohol testing administered in accordance with Part 655 often appears near the beginning of the policy and in conjunction with the list of DOT prohibited substances, as in the Ohio DOT Policy where it appears as a subpoint under prohibited substances (in Section E). Cincinnati Metro covers this requirement under policy (in Part III Section 2.0) immediately before the prohibited substances section. Both the Des Moines MTA and Georgia DOT Policies cover the requirement in the purpose (in Section 2.0) shortly before the prohibited substances section. The statement appears (in Section J) farther from the prohibited substances discussion (Section D) in the Tri-Met Policy. Long Beach Transit covers this requirement in several different areas (in Items 12 through 15 of its policy summary and the introduction to the guidelines).

2.2 Optional Provisions

Employers rarely include optional provisions as a separate section of the policy text. Optional provisions are normally mentioned and identified as additional in the sections where they logically belong. This is the method used in all of the example policies in Appendix A. Some employers use underlines, italics, or bold to distinguish between DOT/FTA (i.e., Parts 40 and 655) and non-DOT/FTA testing requirements. The Cincinnati Metro, Long Beach Transit, and Georgia DOT Policies present the DOT/FTA requirements in bold. The Long Beach Transit and Georgia DOT Policies also italicize the requirements of the Drug-Free Workplace Act of 1988 (49 CFR Part 29). The Ohio DOT Policy uses standard typeface for the DOT/FTA requirements and uses underlines for the transit agency's requirements.

Some employers use a testing notification letter that explicitly informs employees of the authority under which they will be tested. In addition to being clearly differentiated from DOT/FTA requirements, optional provisions should be clearly stated to minimize the likelihood that they will be contested.

Additional requirements often include prohibition and testing of additional substances, employee assistance programs, and rehabilitation options. Most policies prohibit all controlled substances. Some refer to substances prohibited by the Drug Free Workplace Act of 1988. Some employers provide for testing of other substances, e.g., ecstasy, barbiturates, non-barbiturate sedatives (methaqualone), benzodiazipines (Valium, Librium, Xanax), non-amphetamine stimulants, and LSD. LSD is the most difficult and expensive drug to identify forensically. Any additional substances must be listed in the policy if an employer intends to test for them. The Tri-Met Policy (in Section J1a) requires applicants for safety-sensitive positions to provide a second urine specimen for testing of barbiturates, benzodiozepenes, methadone, and propoxyphene. In the Des Moines MTA Policy (in Section 6.0), the MTA "reserves the right" to test, under its own authority, for any drugs that an employee is reasonably suspected of abusing.

2.3 Applicability

Each position title that includes safety-sensitive duties should be listed in the policy regardless of the percentage of the position's duties that are safety sensitive. The policy should also state that all employees and their duties have been reviewed. Including the names of all employees subject to testing is the clearest method, though possibly not practical in organizations with more than a few employees.

Because 85 percent of all court cases related to drug and alcohol testing in the transit industry involve whether the employee testing positive was subject to the testing requirement and why, employers should review all duties and potential duties of each job title and employee. Front-line operations and safety supervisors usually perform safety-sensitive duties. Other managers/ supervisors (e.g., general manager, road supervisor, safety officer, and operations manager) are sometimes considered to be safety-sensitive because they may operate a vehicle. These employees are most likely to operate a vehicle (or perform dispatching duties) at small transit operations that have few employees, where it is often necessary for managers/supervisors to have a broad range of duties, perform multiple roles, or be available to substitute for safety-sensitive employees. Positions that people do not usually think of as being safety-sensitive, such as bus washers, must also be reviewed carefully because the employee may be required to move revenue service vehicles.

The most complicated position to identify as safety-sensitive is dispatcher because the functions vary from agency to agency. According to the FTA definition of safety sensitive, a dispatcher controls movement of vehicles, and in most rail operations and large bus operations this is perfectly clear. However, in many paratransit operations, a dispatcher is merely the person who receives and relays transportation requests or makes schedules. Many of these employers (which are often in rural and small areas) have few appropriate candidates for this position who are willing to be tested. The difficulty is these employees may occasionally be asked to instruct the drivers on routes to destinations.

Employers have stated their applicability policy in a number of ways. Large employers with many positions often use an appendix, attachment, or exhibit to list all safety-sensitive position titles, as in the Cincinnati Metro, Long Beach Transit, and Tri-Met Policies. The Ohio DOT and Georgia DOT Policies, though they are intended for small employers, recommend listing the positions in an attachment. These positions are listed at the end of the Des Moines MTA Policy, following the section on contact persons, but the list is not labeled as an appendix, attachment, or exhibit. Tri-Met also includes the position codes in its list.

Some policies expand applicability beyond the DOT/FTA requirements. Cincinnati Metro, Long Beach Transit, Tri-Met, and Des Moines MTA require all their employees (and applicants) to be tested under the agency's authority for all categories except random. The requirement that non-safety-sensitive employees are also subject to the policy appears near the beginning of the policies (in Part III Section 1.0 of the Cincinnati Metro Policy, in Section III of the Long Beach Transit Guidelines, in Section B of the Tri-Met Policy, and in Section 3.0 of the Des Moines MTA Policy). The exception for random testing in the Tri-Met Policy appears in Section J1d. The exception for random testing in the Des Moines MTA Policy appears in Section 6.0, which also includes an exception for follow-up and return-to-duty testing.

2.4 Prohibited Behavior

The policy should specify behavior prohibited by the employer, including use, manufacture, distribution, dispensing, and possession of controlled substances. Possession and use of alcohol on the premises should also be addressed. Most employers use a separate section for prohibited behavior (or conduct), as in the Tri-Met, Des Moines MTA, Ohio DOT, and Georgia DOT Policies (in Sections E, 5, F, and 5, respectively). Cincinnati Metro, however, addresses this requirement by reprinting the Drug-Free Workplace Act of 1988 in its policy (in Part II). Long Beach Transit cites the prohibited behavior requirements of the Drug-Free Workplace Act for drugs and for alcohol in Items 10 and 21, respectively, of its policy summary.

Another issue to be addressed is use and notification of prescription and over-the-counter drugs. The policy should state that ingestion of controlled substances is prohibited regardless of the source. A procedure for employees to report use of all prescription and over-the-counter drugs and assignment of responsibility for reviewing the reports may be helpful. The Cincinnati Metro Policy addresses use of prescription and over-the-counter drugs under consequences (in Part IV, Section 11.0). Long Beach Transit requires (in Item 9 of its policy summary) employees who take any prescribed medication that could affect their job performance to notify the agency in advance. The Tri-Met Policy requires reporting the use of any legal drugs that may impair performance (in Section H), and mentions use of prescription and over-the-counter drugs under prohibited substances and prohibited behavior (in Sections D and E). The Des Moines MTA, Georgia DOT, and Ohio DOT Policies address use of legal drugs under prohibited substances (in Section 4.2, Section 4.2, and Item 2 of Section E, respectively).

2.5 Testing Circumstances

This section addresses specific issues related to pre-employment, reasonable suspicion, post-accident, and random testing policies. Since return-to-duty and follow-up tests are linked to the employer's consequences policy, they are discussed in Section 2.8.

Some policies address salary compensation for testing. The Des Moines MTA Policy has a subsection (6.1) on compensation for testing. Most employers pay employees' time (including overtime if the testing extends beyond their shift) for all tests except pre-employment (or pre-promotion or transfer), return-to-duty, and follow-up, but often do not state that in their policies. The Des Moines MTA also pays employees' time for follow-up testing. The Cincinnati Metro Policy (in Part III Section 5.6) provides for compensation at the applicable rate for employees during random tests, but compensation is not mentioned under any of the other test categories. The Tri-Met Policy (in Section J1d) requires the employee to be paid overtime for the time that a random test collection extends beyond the end of the shift.

Many policies address payment for re-tests (i.e., split sample) that are performed at the employee's request. Most of them require employees who test positive on split samples to pay for the split sample, though the specifics vary. The Cincinnati Metro Policy (in Part III Section 4.1.3, the Long Beach Transit Guidelines (in Section IXD), and the Ohio DOT Policy (in Section I) require the transit agency to cover the initial cost, but also require the employee to reimburse the agency if the sample is positive. The Des Moines MTA Policy (in Section 6.2) states that all expenses for the test will be collected from the employee via a one-time payroll deduction unless the result invalidates the result of the original test. The Georgia DOT Policy (in Section 6.1, Note 24) recommends including the statement "the split sample test will occur regardless of up-front payment, but that the transit system reserves the right to seek reimbursement from the employee."

Pre-Employment Testing

There are two areas of flexibility in stating the Part 655 requirements for pre-employment testing. First, the employers may, under their own authority, require pre-employment alcohol testing provided their policy states the FTA requirements that pertain to such testing. Second, employers may specify, under their own authority, a shorter time for retesting employees for drugs who have not performed a safety-sensitive function for 90 consecutive days and who have been out of the random test pool during that time.

Reasonable Suspicion Testing

The employer may want to include examples, in the policy, of the legally accepted reasons for ordering reasonable suspicion tests or use wording that the employees are more likely to understand.

Some policies address transportation of employees to the collection site when a reasonable suspicion test is ordered, to ensure they do not drive if unfit (particularly a company vehicle) and that they report immediately and directly to the collection site. The Ohio DOT Policy (in Section L) states "the Transit Department shall be responsible for transporting the employee to the testing site." The Tri-Met Policy (in Section J1b) prohibits the employee from driving home, though the employee is responsible for transportation home; it states that the Transit District will arrange and pay for transportation home if necessary. The Des Moines MTA Policy only states a requirement for employees to be escorted to the collection site under random testing (in Section 6.7), but this requirement is implied for all testing under paid testing (in Section 6.1): ". . . until such time as they are released by the supervisor escorting the employee."

Post-Accident Testing

Some employers provide, in their policy, for testing covered employees for all accidents to remove all decision making of whether to test, which may occur during difficult circumstances. However, they must still decide which authority to test under, and must clearly indicate on the accident report which authority they are testing under. The policy may also use a more stringent definition of an accident, providing it also states the FTA definition. Some employers use a fixed-dollar amount of property damage as the definition. Tri-Met exceeds FTA requirements for post-accident testing. The Tri-Met Policy (in Section J1c) requires a test if an employee receives a citation while on the job for a violation that affects public safety, or violates District rules or procedures and poses a threat to the safety of employees or the public or to property (e.g., a run-away vehicle or allowing a vehicle to strike a fixed object).

Employers may want to address transportation of employees to the collection site when a post-accident test is ordered for the same reasons as addressing it when a reasonable suspicion test is ordered. Transportation is not addressed as frequently for post-accident tests because unfitness for duty is not always suspected as in reasonable suspicion testing. The Tri-Met Policy (in Section J1c) also prohibits the employee from driving home following a post-accident test, though the employee is responsible for transportation home; it states that the Transit District will arrange and pay for transportation home if necessary. The Des Moines MTA Policy implies that employees are to be escorted to the collection site when any drug or alcohol test is ordered, under paid testing (in Section 6.1): ". . . until such time as they are released by the supervisor escorting the employee."

Random Testing

The method used to select safety-sensitive employees for random tests should be stated in the policy. Random-number tables or computer-based random-number generators mapped to safety-sensitive employees' identification numbers are often used.

The FTA testing percentages should also be stated in the policy, and the policy should be modified to reflect FTA adjustments to those percentages.

Employers that choose to test non-DOT/FTA safety-sensitive employees should state in their policy the categories of employees who will be included in their own (non-DOT/FTA) pool, and the rate at which they will be tested. Employers should meet the random test percentages stated in their policies.

Employers may want to require employees selected for random testing to be accompanied by a supervisor to the collection site, to ensure that they report immediately and directly. The Des Moines MTA Policy (in Section 6.7) requires the employee to be escorted immediately to the collection site.

2.6 Testing Methodology and Integrity

The policy need only state that the tests be conducted in accordance with the provisions in 49 CFR Part 40, *Procedures for Federal Workplace Drug and Alcohol Testing Program*. The Tri-Met Policy, in Section J2, states the specimen collection and analysis will be conducted in accordance with U.S. Department of Health and Human Services *Mandatory Guidelines for Federal Workplace Drug Testing Programs, Final Guidelines*, and with Part 40. Many employers, however, repeat portions of the Part 40 Methodology requirements in their policies. This is often done at the request of labor unions. Extensive detail on testing methodology is included, in varying amounts, in the Cincinnati Metro Policy (in Part III Section 4), in the Long Beach Transit Guidelines (in Sections IX, X, XI, and XII), in the Des Moines MTA Policy (in Section 6.0), in the Ohio DOT Policy (in Sections I and J), and in the Georgia DOT Policy (in Section 6.0).

2.7 Refusal Behavior and Consequences

Numerous examples of the behavior that constitutes a refusal to take a drug or alcohol test are listed in Part 40, and in the *Implementation Guidelines*. This information is often incorporated as a separate section (as in the Cincinnati Metro Policy, in Part III Section 7.0) or subsection (as in the Long Beach Transit Guidelines, in Section VIIA3). Long Beach Transit defines refusal under enforcement/ consequences. Another option is to include this information as part of a section on compliance, as in the Tri-Met Policy (in Section I), the Des Moines MTA Policy (in Section 5.4), and the Georgia DOT Policy (in Section 5.4). The Ohio DOT Policy lists numerous examples under its definition of "test refusal" in Section C.

2.8 Consequences of Drug Use and Alcohol Misuse

In addition to stating the minimum consequences required by FTA for violations of the regulations (which are summarized in the *Implementation Guidelines*), the policy should also clearly state the disciplinary action that will be taken by the employer related to the various violations. The disciplinary actions stated in policies and the way that they are stated vary widely.

Some employers (such as Cincinnati Metro and Long Beach Transit) have a zero-tolerance policy for testing positive, or refusing to be tested, for drugs and at 0.04 or higher for alcohol. That is, the employee is terminated for the first offense. Des Moines MTA has a zero-tolerance policy for all positive tests except random, but specifies a second chance for a random positive, though employees testing positive are prohibited from bidding on or driving designated contracted school routes. Many employers state the consequences as discipline up to and including termination, allowing discretion on whether to terminate for a first offense, as in the Tri-Met and Georgia DOT Policies. Tri-Met specifies that the decision will depend on the severity of the violation and the employee's record. The Ohio DOT Policy allows the individual subrecipients to establish their own discipline code. The policy includes all the language and sections needed for a second-chance policy, but has prompts for insertion of "zero tolerance" in the appropriate locations (in Sections A, H, and O).

Experience has shown that consequence/discipline policies that are very specific and allow little discretion tend to receive the fewest legal challenges, particularly in agencies with a strong union presence.

Most employers terminate employees for a first offense of prohibited behavior or for refusing to be tested. Most policies include provisions requiring employees to inform the employer of convictions for drug- and alcohol-related offenses. Most policies also provide lesser consequences for an alcohol test between 0.02

and 0.039, which is not a positive as defined by Part 40. Cincinnati Metro's zero-tolerance policy (in Part IV Section 3.0) allows a second chance for those who test between 0.02 and 0.039 for alcohol, but it requires a disciplinary suspension of at least 30 days without pay (or sick leave) and signing of a last-chance agreement. The Long Beach Transit Guidelines (in Section VIIA1) state that those who test between 0.02 and 0.039 on more than one occasion may be subject to discipline up to and including discharge, but mentions no discipline for the first offense. Both policies offer a second chance for voluntary self-confessors, but require them to complete a rehabilitation program. Most polices exempt self-confessors from disciplinary action and offer treatment opportunities providing they do not test positive. The Des Moines MTA Policy has a separate section (5.8) on voluntary treatment. It requires referral to the SAP at the MTA's expense, but does not require the employee to follow the SAP's recommended treatment plan, though it encourages the employee to do so.

Provisions for grievance and appeal, beyond the FTA protection of MRO review of test results and split-sample testing should also be addressed in the policy. The Tri-Met Policy addresses this issue under discipline (in Section M).

Some policies have separate sections on consequences or discipline, i.e., Long Beach Transit (in Section VIIA of its guidelines), Tri-Met (in Section M), Des Moines MTA (in Section 7.1), and Ohio DOT (in Section Q). In addition to the section on consequences in the Long Beach Transit Guidelines, many of the items (4, 6, 8, 10, 16, 17, 19, 20, and 21) in the Long Beach Transit Policy summary include consequences. The Tri-Met Policy also discusses consequences under prohibited behavior (in Section E) and under return to work (in Section N). The Des Moines MTA Policy also discusses consequences in various subsections under prohibited conduct (in Section 5), under return-to-duty testing (in Section 6.8), and under re-entry conditions (in Section 8.0). The Ohio DOT Policy includes a note for zero-tolerance employers to remove the provisions that specify discipline other than termination. The Cincinnati Metro Policy has a separate part (IV) on consequences with separate sections on 11 categories of violations. The Georgia DOT Policy covers consequences under treatment requirements (in Section 5.5) and under test procedures (in Section 6.0).

The placement of the requirement that all employees who test positive be referred to a SAP varies from policy to policy. This requirement appears in a separate section on SAP referral in the Cincinnati Metro, Long Beach Transit, and Tri-Met Polices. The SAP referral section is under rehabilitation (in Part V Section 2.0) in the Cincinnati Metro Policy, in Section XII of the Long Beach Transit Guidelines, and under general provisions for drug and alcohol testing (in Section J3) in the Tri-Met Policy. The requirement is included under compliance with testing requirements in the Des Moines MTA Policy (in Section 6.0), under result of drug/alcohol test in the Ohio DOT Policy (in Section Q), and under testing procedures in the Georgia DOT Policy (in Section 6.0).

Return-to-Duty and Follow-Up Testing

All policies that allow a second chance must discuss return-to-duty and follow-up testing. Because "zero-tolerance" policies often have exceptions for self-confessors or for alcohol tests under 0.04 (e.g., the Cincinnati Metro and Long Beach Transit Policies), all employers should address return-to-duty and follow-up testing in their policy. Both the Cincinnati Metro Policy and the Long Beach Transit Guidelines include sections on return-to-duty and follow-up testing (in Part III Sections 5.3 and 5.4 and in Section VIIIE, respectively) and on rehabilitation (in Part V Section 3.0 and in Section XIII, respectively). Even an employer that requires termination for all first violations and gives no grace for self-confessors should include these provisions in case it is required to reinstate an employee, by a higher authority such as the Fair Labor Relations Board.

Most employers require the employee, or the employee's insurance carrier, to pay for rehabilitation and the required return-to-duty and follow-up tests. These requirements should be included in the policy and identified as independent of FTA authority. All of the policies in Appendix A require the employee to be responsible for treatment and rehabilitation cost.

2.9 Designated Contact Person

Although this requirement is listed first in the policy-content requirements, Part 655 does not specify where in the policy to include the identity of the contact person. Most employers include it at the end of the policy, as in the Tri-Met, Des Moines MTA, Ohio DOT, and Georgia DOT examples. (Tri-Met includes its contact persons under program administration, in Section P.) However, some employers include the name on the first page. Long Beach Transit includes the contact person on the first page of its guidelines, in Section II. Still others place it in an appendix along with the names and contact information for other important professionals and vendors (e.g., MROs, SAPs, collection sites, and laboratories), as in the Cincinnati Metro Policy (in Appendix B). Long Beach Transit includes an extended list of contacts in an attachment, in addition to the contact name on the first page of the guidelines. An appendix or attachment provides employees with a "quick reference guide" to this information, and it enables distribution of a revised appendix or attachment with updated contact information, thereby avoiding the need to re-adopt and redistribute the policy.

The person designated to answer employee questions about the drug and alcohol program is often the person responsible for program administration. For smaller organizations, this may be a human resources manager, an operations manager, or a general manager. The contact person's position title, address, telephone number, and fax number should also be included, as well as the words "and their successor."

3. Education and Training

This chapter discusses methods for meeting the FTA education and training requirements contained in Part 655.14, as discussed in the *Implementation Guidelines* (in Chapter 5). The issues related to meeting those requirements are also discussed.

3.1 Education

Informational materials on prohibited drug use include posters, pamphlets and brochures, fact sheets, and newsletter articles. These materials are often distributed to new employees with orientation materials, and are communicated via postings and displays in common areas of the workplace, anti-drug abuse campaigns, and seminars. A common source of these materials is employee assistance programs (EAPs).

Many transit agencies have contracts with EAP providers to assist employees with various types of personal problems. These contracts often require the EAP to supply and distribute educational materials on substance abuse. EAPs often issue brochures and posters to employers and mail informational materials directly to employees' homes. EAPs also provide employees with evaluation and referral, short-term individual counseling, individual case management, crisis intervention (24-hour crisis line), and employee educational programs.

The Center for Substance Abuse Prevention provides EAP models, as well as telephone information and literature on policy, drug testing, and related topics, at no cost to employers. It also provides referrals to other information sources and lists of consultants by geographic area. This information can be received or ordered through the Center's Drug-Free Workplace Help line, (800) 843-497, between 9:00 a.m. and 8:00 p.m. EST Monday through Friday.

Other national organizations that are frequently used as sources of educational information and materials include:

- Americans for a Drug-Free America--This organization distributes various pamphlets on the effects of illegal drug use. These materials are published by American Crisis Publishing, Inc., 3800 Hudson Bend Road, Austin, TX 78734, (512) 266-2485.

- National Safety Alliance (NSA), P.O. Box 159060, Nashville, TN 37215, (615) 832-0046--Many transit agencies distribute the NSA handbook titled *Substance Abuse Training for the Workplace.*

- National Clearinghouse for Alcohol and Drug Information (NCADI), P.O. Box 2345, Rockville, MD 20852, (800) 729-6686, (301) 468-2600--The Clearinghouse provides fact sheets, films, posters, pamphlets, and brochures at no or low cost. Multilingual materials and a free quarterly catalog are also available.

- Partnership for a Drug Free America, 405 Lexington Avenue, New York, NY 10174-0002, (212) 922-1560—This organization provides posters, audiotapes, and videotapes with high-impact messages. There is no charge for these materials, but donations are requested.

Health insurance carriers, mental health agencies, and state substance abuse clearinghouses also provide informational and educational materials on substance abuse for distribution to employers. Each State has at least one federally funded clearinghouse that provides nationally and locally produced materials.

3.2 Training

Various approaches and combinations of approaches are used to meet both of the training requirements in Part 655.14(b). Some employers use one approach or combination to train their safety-sensitive employees and another one to train their supervisors and other company officials who are responsible for determining reasonable suspicion of drug and alcohol use.

Most of these approaches involve some type of classroom training with an instructor or facilitator leading the session. The most comprehensive approach includes a lecture, presentation of a video, or use of some other interactive technology, a question-and-answer session, discussion of the company policy and issues relevant to the employer's operation, and role playing. A professional on the effects and indications of substance abuse would give the lecture, show the video, and answer questions about substance abuse. A person knowledgeable about the employer's operations (e.g., a human resources official, drug and alcohol program manager (DAPM), or a third-party administrator (TPA)--would answer questions about the employer's operations and lead discussions related to the work environment. In some cases, one person can perform both functions, such as a DAPM who is also a health professional or a TPA who is a substance abuse consultant.

Many large and medium-size employers and consortia contract with consulting firms experienced in delivering workplace training or other substance abuse professionals to prepare a curriculum and present it. Some of these large organizations have a professional on their internal staff or a TPA who prepares or presents the curriculum. Sometimes the internal professional or TPA presents a curriculum prepared by a consulting firm or contracted professionals. In some cases, internal professionals work with consultants or contractors to prepare and present the training.

Smaller entities not affiliated with a consortium often have a staff member lead the training using commercial training programs or training manuals and materials acquired from their state department of transportation (DOT), a nearby transit agency, or FTA. Self-paced training programs in booklet and videotape formats are available from standard suppliers of training materials for the transit industry or from companies and individuals that advertise on the Internet. Some state DOTs purchase these materials and distribute them to their transit employers, particularly for small entities with limited budgets. Other state DOTs hire consultants to prepare standard training manuals (or prepare them using internal staff) for their transit agencies.

Discussion and role-playing techniques can be used with any of these approaches at minimal additional expense, and are very effective because they allow the agency's staff to address other issues.

Professionals who may prepare training curricula or provide training include:
- EAP providers
- Nurses and physicians
- Mental health professionals
- Drug and alcohol treatment specialists
- Pharmacists
- Toxicologists
- Law enforcement drug awareness specialists

Organizations that may be sources for identifying or locating training professionals include:
- National organizations and their local affiliates, such as the Employee Assistance Professionals Association and their state chapters and the National Council on Alcoholism and Drug Dependence
- State substance abuse clearinghouses
- State-wide nonprofit organizations, such as Connecticut's "Drugs Don't Work!" or Texas' "War on Drugs"

Though FTA requires that all training records be kept for only 2 years, many employers retain all training records indefinitely. This is particularly important if consulting companies or contracted professionals are used.

Training for Safety-Sensitive Employees

The required drug abuse training is often incorporated in the employee orientation process. Many employers find it difficult to cover all the required information in 60 minutes, particularly if questions, discussions, and role playing are included. Some trainers also test the participants before they begin to assess their knowledge and enable them to tailor the training to the employees' needs. They may also test them again upon completion to asses their comprehension. Thus, many transit agencies have found 2 hours to be a more appropriate drug training period. It is also helpful to encourage employees to talk to their physicians and supervisors about over-the-counter and prescription medications to determine alternatives to their use while on duty. Some employers also cover alcohol misuse and aspects of drug abuse not required by Part 655.14, such as effects of additional illegal drugs and over-the-counter and prescription medications.

Videos are a useful tool for employee training, providing they support and do not contradict the specifics of the FTA regulations. One example of an effective video is *Effects of Drugs and Alcohol on the Human Body* by Comdata, though FTA does not endorse the product.

The Florida Department of Transportation has a Public Transportation Substance Abuse Program that it distributes to the FTA grantees in Florida. The Employee's Manual and Instructor's Manual will be available on the FTA Office of Safety and Security website: http://transit-safety.volpe.dot.gov. The program contains modules on:

- Drugs and public safety
- Alcohol
- Each of the FTA prohibited drugs
- Over-the-counter drugs
- Combining drugs
- Florida DOT policy
- Availability of help
- A test and certification

The Des Moines Metropolitan Transit Authority (MTA) has a *Substance Abuse Training Manual*, which will also be available on the FTA Office of Safety and Security website: http://transit-safety.volpe.dot.gov. This manual addresses:

- The Regulatory Requirements
- Jobs considered Safety Sensitive
- Required Types of Testing

- Signs, Symptoms, and Effects of the Five Prohibited Drugs
- Alcohol Testing
- Sample Collection Procedures
- Role of Outside Professionals and Hotline Telephone Number
- Confidentiality
- Disciplinary Action

The Des Moines MTA Training Manual also includes the outline for the training for safety-sensitive employees:

Des Moines MTA Substance Abuse Training Outline

- Impact of Drug Abuse on Society and Industry
  - National, Regional, and Local Statistics on Prohibited Drug Use
  - Safety, Personal Health, and Work Environment
- Response of the Federal Government and the Transit Industry
  - Drug-Free Workplace Act
  - Prevention of Alcohol Misuse and Prohibited Drug Use in Transit Operations (49 CFR Part 655)
  - Procedures for Transportation Workplace Drug and Alcohol Testing Programs (49 CFR Part 40)
  - MTA Policy on Prohibited Drugs and Alcohol
- Safety, Personal Health, and Work Environment Effects of Each of the Five Prohibited Drugs
- Manifestations and Behavioral Cues That May Indicate Use of Each of the Five Prohibited Drugs
- Procedures and Protections of the FTA Drug and Alcohol Testing Program
- Questions and Answers

When hiring professional trainers, employers should be sure that the trainers thoroughly understand the FTA regulations. The same caution should be exercised when acquiring self-paced training materials. Many trainers and training material producers prepare and deliver products used to comply with the Federal Motor Carrier Safety Administration (FMCSA) requirements, and believe that they also apply to FTA. The FMCSA and FTA regulations have significant differences. Applying the FMCSA requirements to a transit program could affect employer liability and employee civil rights.

Important criteria to consider in selecting a trainer are:

- Workplace experience with transit or similar industries
- Concern with safety, cost reduction, productivity, liability, and public image, as well as employee welfare
- Understanding of Parts 40 and 655 and how to respond to employee attitudes and concerns regarding drug and alcohol testing

- Training style, platform skills, techniques, tools, and methods appropriate to adult learning, including appropriate and high-quality audio/visual material, handouts, role playing, and case studies

- Willingness to learn about the customer's operations, policy, programs, values, and culture

- Flexibility, professionalism, and tact in handling diverse opinions and needs of resistant employees, assertive managers, supervisors, executives, and union representatives

Some professional trainers use commercial off-the-shelf curricula. Such curricula have to be tailored to reflect the employer's procedures, discipline policy, and EAP. The employer may want to have its own human resources, medical, or labor relations professional work with the contracted training professionals in developing and presenting the training sessions.

Training for Determining Reasonable Suspicion of Drug and Alcohol Abuse

Most employers exceed the scope of the requirements in Part 655(2)(b). Additional topics typically addressed in supervisory training include:

- Role and responsibility of supervisors and other company officials who are responsible for determining reasonable suspicion

- Initiating, substantiating, and documenting a test referral

- Intervention and confrontation with employees

Other elements that can further improve the training effectiveness include introducing the context of the regulation, reviewing the testing program requirements, and reviewing agency disciplinary procedures. Role playing has proved to be especially effective in reasonable suspicion training.

Given their tendency to expand the scope, most employers have found that reasonable suspicion cannot be effectively covered in the required minimum of 60 minutes. A comprehensive program often requires 3 hours of training for drugs and an additional 3 hours for alcohol. Medium-size and large transit agencies often dedicate at least a day or two to reasonable suspicion training. The Massachusetts Bay Transportation Authority (MBTA), for example, has developed a week-long program for determining reasonable suspicion of drug and alcohol use. The MBTA program consists of live presentations and extensive role playing, and is presented by contracted professional trainers, the MBTA Medical Unit, and the EAP provider. Considerable research and effort has been spent on developing the program, based on the environment at the MBTA. In the past, the agency experimented with commercial off-the-shelf presentations and videotaping of MBTA materials, and found both approaches to be far less effective than live presentations.

Because identification of suspicious behavior is an important part of a substance abuse prevention program and it is difficult and uncomfortable for many supervisors, many employers require refresher training at specified intervals.

A video and a leader's guide on reasonable suspicion have been produced for and are available from FTA at no charge. The video consists of four segments:

    (1) General Requirements on Reasonable Suspicion Referrals

    (2) Alcohol Abuse in the Workplace

    (3) Prohibited Drug Use in the Workplace

    (4) Make the Call: the Reasonable Suspicion Interview

The Leader's Guide —*Reasonable Suspicion Referral for Drug and Alcohol Testing: A Training Program for Transit Supervisors, Leader's Guide*— will be available on the FTA Office of Safety and Security website: http://transit-safety.volpe.dot.gov. It contains a trainer packet and a trainee packet on five exercises:

    (1) General Requirements for Making Reasonable Suspicion Referrals

    (2) Alcohol Abuse in the Workplace

    (3) Prohibited Drug Use in the Workplace

    (4) Make the Call: the Reasonable Suspicion Interview

    (5) Wrap-up Discussion

The Hartford (Connecticut) Regional Transit District has documented its supervisor training in a manual (prepared by NSA) titled *Substance Abuse in the Workplace: Supervisor Training.* This manual, which is used by all but one of the approximately 60 transit operators in the state, addresses the following issues: identification of a problem, the supervisor's role in an effective substance abuse program, situations confronting supervisors, reasonable suspicion testing information and step processes, and three parts of an effective confrontation interview. It also contains appendices on drug retention time in the body and suggested demeanor for supervisors, tips on confrontational interviews, documentation forms, and DOT information.

The Des Moines MTA *Substance Abuse Training Manual* (mentioned in the discussion of training for safety-sensitive employees) also includes the outline for the MTA's additional training for supervisors and other officials responsible for determining reasonable suspicion:

Des Moines MTA Reasonable Suspicion Training Outline

- Impact of Drug Abuse on Society and Industry
  - National, Regional, and Local Statistics on Prohibited Drug Use
  - Safety, Personal Health, and Work Environment
- Response of the Federal Government and the Transit Industry
  - Drug-Free Workplace Act
  - Prevention of Alcohol Misuse and Prohibited Drug Use in Transit Operations (49 CFR Part 655)
  - Procedures for Transportation Workplace Drug and Alcohol Testing Programs (49 CFR Part 40)
  - MTA Policy on Prohibited Drugs and Alcohol
- Safety, Personal Health, and Work Environment Effects of Alcohol Use and Prohibited Drug Use
- Procedures and Protections of the MTA Drug and Alcohol Testing Program
- Responsibility of Supervisors, Especially as Related to Drug and Alcohol Programs
  - To Supervise
  - To Deal with Problems in Workplace (e.g., Unacceptable, Deteriorating, and Unsafe Performance)
- Indicators of Probable Alcohol Misuse or Prohibited Drug Misuse (common to all substance abuse and individually to alcohol and to each of the 5 DOT prohibited drugs)
  - Physical
  - Behavioral
  - Speech
  - Performance
  - Body Odors
- Supervisory Responsibilities Related to Reasonable Suspicion
  - Removal from Safety-Sensitive Position
  - Observation and Documentation
  - Confidentiality of the Employee
  - Review Findings
  - Make Reasonable Suspicion Decision
  - Escort to Collection Site
  - Escort Home
  - Special Considerations in Dealing with Alcohol- or Drug-Influenced Employees
- Conflict Resolution
- Resources Available to the Supervisor
  - Drug and Alcohol Program Manager (DAPM) and Designated Employer Representative (DER)
  - Medical Review Officer
  - Substance Abuse Professional
  - Employee Assistance Program
  - Security and Law Enforcement
  - Other
- Questions and Answers

---

4. Testing Program Implementation and Management

The employer is ultimately responsible for maintaining an FTA mandated Drug and Alcohol Testing Program that complies with 49 CFR Parts 40 and 655. Likewise, the grantee is responsible for ensuring that all of its operations and maintenance contractors and subrecipients maintain a compliant program. The required program consists of three test functions: urine collection and analysis, breath collection and analysis, and medical review.

Each employer must have an employee or employees responsible for ensuring operation of a compliant program. Large employers often have a separate position for administering the program, often referred to as Drug and Alcohol Program Manager (DAPM) and occasionally as Substance Abuse Program Manager (SAPM). The responsibilities of this position are sometimes performed by more than one employee. Small employers do not usually have a separate position of DAPM or SAPM; the program management functions are assigned to an employee or employees to perform in addition to their other duties.

Program managers come from various backgrounds, and there is no particular discipline that seems to provide a more appropriate experience than any other. The most common backgrounds include general manager, operations management, safety, risk management, human resources, and administrative assistant. The primary requirement is that they are very knowledgeable of the regulations; all employees who perform program management functions should attend FTA seminars conducted by the Transportation Safety Institute (TSI).

Some employers use their employees to perform all the program management functions while others hire third party administrators (TPA) to administer part or all of their program. The three test functions are frequently contracted out, though some large employers use internal staff to perform one or two or all three of these functions. Employers must have an effective overarching method for ensuring that the required tests are performed in accordance with the policy and records are kept.

This chapter addresses the issues associated with implementing and maintaining a compliant program and references best practice examples (contained in Appendices B, C, D, and E) for addressing them. These discussions appear in five sections:

(1) **Internal administration** (managing DAPM functions performed by the employer's staff, examples in Appendix B)

(2) **External administration** (procuring service agents and monitoring service agents and contractors/subrecipients, examples in Appendix C)

(3) **Specimen collection and analysis** (both urine and breath, examples in Appendix D)

(4) **Medical review** (examples in Appendix E)

(5) **Records management**

4.1 Internal Administration

This section addresses general administrative issues and concerns and the issues related to and methods used for ensuring compliance with the four types of testing required for all employers: pre-employment, reasonable suspicion, post-accident, and random. (Issues related to return-to-duty and follow-up tests are discussed in Chapter 5.) Though this section may be most useful to program managers who either perform the functions themselves or delegate them to internal staff, the discussions here and the examples in Appendix B may also be useful to managers who contract out their administrative functions. They can be used as benchmarks or standards in evaluating performance of TPAs and can be offered as advice or tools to TPAs and contractors/subrecipients.

Many employers use forms and checklists to create consistent routines for performing administrative functions and to document completion of those functions. Appendix B contains examples that have been used successfully.

General Administrative Duties

A frequent audit finding is no evidence that employees received the policy statement. Some grantees require that safety-sensitive employees sign forms acknowledging that they have received the drug and alcohol policy statement, and retain the documents as a means of proof of notification. Examples of policy receipt certification forms used by the Massachusetts Bay Transportation Authority (MBTA), the Washington Metropolitan Area Transportation Authority (WMATA), and the Tri-County Metropolitan Transit Authority (Tri-Met), Portland, OR, appear in Figures B-1, B-2, and B-3, respectively.

Lists of employees and supervisors, or other company officials, who attend and complete required training are often maintained to provide documentation that the training requirement was met. Lists used by Cincinnati Metro for this purpose appear in Figures B-4 and B-5, respectively. Some employers also issue certificates to each employee who completes the training, and retain file copies of the certificates issued. Figure B-6 is a an example of a form, used by the Government of the Virgin Islands, for certifying that supervisors or other company officials have received the required reasonable suspicion training.

The City of Albuquerque uses printed lists to document and disseminate the roles and responsibilities of the Program Manager, department program coordinators, departmental divisional contacts, and front-line supervisors, shown in Figures B-7, B-8, B-9, and B-10, respectively.

The City of Albuquerque also uses an Excel spread sheet with tracking facility as a master log to assist with managing each of the four types of FTA tests required for all employers. These are discussed and referenced individually later in this section under their respective testing types. The MBTA uses a single log, shown in Figure B-11, to track all testing.

The City of Albuquerque uses a form (shown in Figure B-12) to document the results of each test through each step of the process, from collection to the disciplinary action. This form includes provision for signatures by the laboratory scientists who identify the result and the medical review officer (MRO) who reviews it.

Broward County (Florida) Transit provides a log (shown in Figure B-13) for each supervisor to fill out whenever a test is ordered. This form provides for a very detailed sequence of events. It allows the employer to monitor the amount of time the employee spends en route to the site, the amount of time spent waiting to be tested after arriving at the site, and the amount of time the employee spends on the return trip to work.

Forms are commonly used to notify employees of ordered tests and to document the order. Notification forms used by the Ohio Department of Transportation (DOT) and MV Transportation (an operations contractor for several transit agencies) appear in Figures B-14 and B-15, respectively. The MV Transportation form includes the time that the employee is sent for testing and the time the employee arrives at the collection site, and it provides for transportation to the site by a supervisor.

Forms are also used to document and notify management of positive test results. Figures B-16 and B-17 are forms used by the Los Angeles County Metropolitan Transportation Authority (LACMTA) to document positive drug test results and positive alcohol test results, respectively. The MBTA uses one form (shown in Figure B-18) to notify an employee of a positive drug or alcohol result. The MBTA also uses a form (shown in Figure B-19) to notify the immediate supervisor of an employee's positive result.

Pre-Employment Testing

The West Virginia DOT Division of Public Transit documents its pre-employment testing process in a flow chart, shown in Figure B-20.

The City of Albuquerque uses a summary sheet (shown in Figure B-21) to document the test of each applicant for a safety-sensitive position, including both FTA and City definitions of safety sensitive. Albuquerque's Excel spreadsheet master log for tracking pre-employment testing appears in Figure B-22.

The MBTA uses a form (shown in Figure B-23) to notify an applicant for a safety-sensitive position of a positive drug or alcohol result.

Reasonable Suspicion Testing

The West Virginia DOT Division of Public Transit documents its reasonable suspicion testing process in a flow chart, shown in Figure B-24. Western Maine Transportation Services, a small rural seasonal fixed-route bus system, documents its reasonable suspicion testing process in a slightly different flow chart and uses a form along with it to document symptoms and referrals, as shown in Figure B-25.

Three variations on documentation forms used by large systems appear in Figures B-26, B-27, and B-28—LACMTA, MBTA, and Albuquerque, respectively. Ohio DOT also distributes the form shown Figure B-28 to its subrecipients, which include many small systems. The LACMTA form is the most compact of the three and calls for the least amount of written explanation.

Both the San Francisco Bay Area Rapid Transit (BART) District and the Denver Regional Transit District (RTD) use a single form to document circumstances for ordering both reasonable suspicion and post-accident tests. BART's "Observation/Incident Report" appears in Figure B-29, and Denver RTD's "Accident/Incident/Reasonable Cause Report" appears in Figure B-30. Both forms distinguish between tests ordered per FTA authority and those ordered under the transit district's rules. The BART form lists the criteria for testing under each set of rules separately, and lists BART's procedures for reasonable suspicion testing on the back of the form, along with a space for comments, incident description, and action taken. The Denver form requires the supervisor to check which rules apply to the test ordered, but does not describe the rules. The Denver form is the only one of the six aforementioned reasonable suspicion documentation forms that does not require the supervisor to check off observed behavioral and appearance symptoms from an extensive list. It requires written comments under several different categories. The groupings of symptoms used in the six different examples vary widely.

Albuquerque also requires its supervisors to fill out and sign a summary report (shown in Figure B-31) for each reasonable suspicion test ordered, in addition to filling out the "Fitness for Duty" form shown in Figure B-28. Albuquerque's

Excel spreadsheet master log for tracking reasonable suspicion testing is shown in Figure B-32.

Occasionally, a reasonable suspicion test ordered by a supervisor is not administered. It is useful to document these occasions on a standard form. Albuquerque's summary report (shown in Figure B-31) has a block for explaining such an occurrence. Sioux Falls Transit System (SuTran), South Dakota, uses a separate form (shown in Figure B-33) when an ordered reasonable suspicion drug test is not performed.

Many times, employees have tested negative in FTA reasonable suspicion tests even though the criteria for ordering the tests was met. Employers should understand that many of the symptoms that are basis for these tests are also symptoms of other problems (e.g., marital stress, sleep disorders, job dissatisfaction) that may impair performance of safety-sensitive functions. Though it is not required by FTA, some employers require (or strongly recommend) counseling for employees who test negative in properly ordered reasonable suspicion tests, to identify such problems.

Post-Accident Testing

Many employers have devised forms to assist supervisors in determining whether to test operators following an accident (and under what authority), in documenting procedures to be followed after the decision is made, in recording all the required information, and in providing explanations of why tests were not conducted at specific times.

The Greater Cleveland Regional Transit Authority (GCRTA) issues a two-sided card (shown in Figure B-34) to its supervisors. The front side contains a decision tree for determining whether to order a post-accident test under FTA authority. The back lists the criteria for ordering a test under GCRTA authority. However, the GCRTA card is merely a decision-making guide; it requires no documentation.

The West Virginia DOT Division of Public Transit documents its post-testing process in a flow chart shown in Figure B-35. It also issues a decision-making form (shown in Figure B-36) for supervisors to fill out to document occurrences and decisions made following each accident. It requires the supervisor to note which authority (FTA or company) the decision to test was made under, and to explain why an alcohol test was not performed within 8 hours of the accident and a drug test was not performed within 32 hours of the accident.

The San Francisco BART "Observation/Incident Report" (shown in Figure B-29) requires supervisors to check off post-accident criteria that are met following an accident. There are two lists of three items each—one list with FTA criteria and the other with BART criteria. A test should be ordered if any of the items are checked; it should be an FTA test if any FTA item is checked. This BART report also requires the supervisor to check off symptoms, from the extensive list, observed in the operator following the accident. The presence of these symptoms could be basis for ordering a reasonable suspicion test if none of the post-accident criteria are met. BART also issues procedural instructions (shown in Figure B-37) to be followed when an accident occurs. These include making the decision and what to do after either decision is made.

The Denver RTD "Accident/Incident/Reasonable Cause Report" (shown in Figure B-30) requires written explanations under the three FTA non-fatal-accident test scenarios, completion of the reasonable cause section if the second or third scenario exists, and indication of whether FTA or RTD rules apply. The FTA post-accident test criteria are listed on the back of the form.

LACMTA uses a form (shown in Figure B-38) that summarizes the FTA post-accident testing regulations, and requires the supervisor to document answers to questions leading to a decision of whether to test under FTA authority, requires documentation of reasons why tests are delayed or not performed if FTA criteria are met, and provides a checklist of procedures.

Figures B-39 and B-40 also show forms that require complete documentation of accident information, including whether ordered tests were performed at specific times with explanations if they were not performed. Figure B-39 is used by the Southeastern Pennsylvania Transportation Authority (SEPTA). It provides a checklist of both FTA and SEPTA criteria. Figure B-40 is a summary report that the City of Albuquerque requires its supervisors to complete and submit within 24 hours of an accident. SuTran uses a separate form (shown in Figure B-41) when an FTA criterion for a post-accident test is met but no test is performed within 32 hours.

Figure B-42 is Albuquerque's Excel spreadsheet master log for tracking post-accident testing.

Random Testing

Figures B-43 and B-44 are flow charts showing procedures for random testing. The two charts use different approaches. The approach in Figure B-43, which is used by the West Virginia DOT Division of Public Transit, is oriented to the employee's response to the testing order. There are two separate event sequences following the notification of testing: one for the employees who report to the collection site as ordered and another for those who do not report. There are also two separate sequences for employees who report to the collection site: one for those who provide a specimen and another for those who do not. The approach in Figure B-44, which is used by San Francisco BART, is oriented to the supervisor who is notified of an employee's selection. It lists the steps to be followed by the supervisor.

Many employers notify their employees of selection for a random test in writing, and keep copies of the notices in their records. Figures B-45 and B-46, used by BART and the MBTA, respectively, are examples of notices of selection for a random test. Both of these forms call for documentation of all pertinent notification information, contain instructions to the selected employee chosen for a random test and consequences for non-compliance, and require the employee to sign the form to acknowledge receipt.

The City of Albuquerque has a comprehensive set of forms that it uses to disseminate instructions and provide for documentation of its random selection process. The instructions for the selections process are listed in Figure B-47. The roles and responsibilities of the selector are listed in Figure B-48. The form used by the Transit Department to list the names of all the employees selected during a particular draw appears in Figure B-49; this list includes the date and time of the scheduled test, the test notification, and the actual test. A separate form, shown in Figure B-50, is used to list all employees within each department tested during each test period and to record their collection dates and times. The form used to document each individual test order, the result, and the action taken when the result is positive appears in Figure B-51. Figure B-52 is Albuquerque's Excel spreadsheet master log for tracking random testing.

Excel spreadsheets with a tracking facility have proved especially useful in tracking random testing.

Forms can also be used to help employers keep the random pool fully populated with all currently working employees. The Rhode Island Public Transit Authority (RIPTA) requires that an employee status form, shown in Figure B-53, be filled out whenever a safety-sensitive employee begins or terminates work. This form is used to add or delete the employee's name from the random pool.

4.2 External Administration

As previously mentioned, many employers contract out some or all of their administrative responsibilities to TPAs. Small transit agencies and operations and maintenance contractors often enter into a TPA consortium (C/TPA) with other small employers, for economic and logistical reasons. Larger agencies and contractors often hire their own TPAs. Administrative functions performed by TPAs vary widely from employer to employer and consortium to consortium. TPAs are sometimes used to procure and monitor other service agents—urine collectors and laboratories, screen test technicians (STTs) and breath analysis technicians (BATs), medical review officers (MROs), and substance abuse professionals (SAPs). Some TPAs even employ some or all of these specialists on their staff. Many employers, however, contract with these service agents directly.

Program managers should exercise caution when selecting service agents. Some of the large nationwide companies, particularly TPAs, have the worst compliance records. Program managers also need to closely and proactively monitor all of their contracted service agents, as well as the programs conducted by any subrecipients or operations and maintenance contractors subject to Parts 40 and 655.

Procurement of Service Agents

Many employers seek service agents that are part of a trade association. Membership is no guarantee of a quality provider, but it is an advantage. The members are informed, some associations have a certification process, and substandard performance and uncooperative behavior by member providers can be reported to the organization. Examples of these organizations include:

- Drug & Alcohol Testing Industry Association: 800-355-1257, www.datia.org

- American Association of Medical Review Officers: 919-489-5407

- American Society of Addictive Medicine: 301-656-3920

- American College of Occupational and Environmental Medicine: 847-228-6850

- Substance Abuse Program Administration Association: 800-672-7229

The following general steps have proved helpful in selecting various types of service agents for FTA drug and alcohol testing programs. These steps apply to all providers:

- Contact other employers in the area to identify vendors that have performed their duties well. (Either local or nationwide companies can be suitable.)

- Prepare a written request for proposals (RFP) that clearly states the procedures that must be effectively performed by each type of provider needed, including complete documentation of their professional credentials, a short statement on the FTA procedures for their specialty and how they contrast with other applications they have been involved with, and a summary of the training that their personnel have received and how their performance is monitored.

- Formulate standards for evaluating the proposals, assemble a panel to review the proposals against the standards, select those that score the highest on the evaluation, and invite them for a brief presentation of their proposal and a question and answer session.

- Formulate a checklist of questions for the interview that will demonstrate their understanding of the relevant FTA requirements and will reveal the training received by their personnel for all functions to be performed.

- Take detailed notes during the interviews so the data can be used in the final evaluation process by the evaluation panel.

- Select the agency that scores the highest.

- Enter an agreement that, ideally, includes a provision allowing the transit agency to terminate the contract at will and for convenience.

Specific advice for selecting specimen collection and analysis companies, MROs, and SAPs appear in Section 4.3, Section 4.4, and Chapter 5, respectively.

Oversight of Service Agents and Contractors/Subrecipients

To help ensure that contracted service agents comply with the regulations, many employers develop a relationship with their providers. They talk with them, ask questions, impose performance standards, require documentation, visit their facilities at least once per year to perform informal reviews or formal audits, and impose corrective action for non-compliance. Employers can also report substandard performance and uncooperative behavior by service agents to FTA. If problems persist, FTA can initiate a Public Interest Exclusion (PIE), under Part 40, against the service vendor.

Because grantees (and other employers) are responsible for the compliance of their operations and maintenance contractors and all subrecipients, they often develop similar relationships with those entities as developed with service agents. Many grantees also require quarterly management reports summarizing test reports and annual management information systems (MIS) reports.

The *Implementation Guidelines* contain regulatory checklists for evaluating compliance of service agents and contractors/subrecipients. Appendix C contains examples of forms and lists used by state DOTs and transit agencies for monitoring compliance of subrecipients, operations and maintenance contractors, and contracted service agents.

Minnesota DOT issues comprehensive checklists to its subrecipients for monitoring their TPAs and C/TPAs, shown in Figures C-1 and C-2, respectively. Specific issues and concerns related to monitoring specimen collection and analysis companies, MROs, and SAPs appear in Section 4.3, Section 4.4, and Chapter 5, respectively.

LACMTA issues written guidelines, shown in Figure C-3, to all of its operations and maintenance contractors. These guidelines are used as a basis for judging compliance when LACMTA staff visit the contractor's facilities. GCRTA uses a single-page form, shown in Figure C-4, for documenting compliance when its staff visit the contractor's facilities. Ohio DOT uses a very detailed multi-page checklist, shown in Figure C-5, for evaluating the programs of contractors.

4.3 Specimen Collection and Analysis

Many of the concerns and issues associated with urine collection and breath collection are similar, and both tests are often ordered at the same time and performed at the same facility. Therefore, this section addresses both of these functions. It is organized by the following topics: collection procedures, collection facilities, monitoring of collection and analysis operations, and selection of collection and analysis service agents. Within each topic, issues that are unique to each collection process are discussed separately. The analysis procedures are different and are also discussed separately. Examples of forms and lists used to assist with specimen collection appear in Appendix D.

Collection Procedures

As mentioned in Chapter 2, some transit agencies require, in their policies, that employees ordered to take reasonable suspicion or post-accident tests be transported or escorted to the collection site to ensure that they travel directly to the site. Transporting or escorting people for all tests is good practice, if feasible, and can be required when the test is ordered even if the requirement is not documented in the policy.

As in all aspects of the testing process, forms can be a useful tool in communicating collection practices and documenting occurrences, such as arrival times and performance of the various steps in the process. San Francisco BART issues collection instructions (shown in Figure D-1) to each employee who is tested, and requires urine collectors to complete and sign a checklist (shown in Figure D-2) for each collection performed.

Forms are also useful in documenting a donor's inability, or unwillingness, to produce a urine or breath specimen. Ohio DOT issues "shy bladder" and "shy lung" forms (shown in Figures D-3 and D-4, respectively) to its subrecipients to document these occurrences. Some delays in producing specimens by donors who ultimately produce a negative specimen have been interpreted as a ploy to collect additional pay or avoid work. A useful device for monitoring the amount of water consumed by "shy bladder" donors is to issue 10-ounce bottles of water one at a time to a maximum of four bottles, record the number of empty bottles, and observe the consumption.

Another frequent issue in urine collection is hand washing. Many donors do not want to handle their own pen before they wash their hands and do not want to use the collector's pen that was used by others before they washed their hands. One solution is to issue throw-away pens.

Collection Facilities

Some large transit authorities, such as New York City Transit (NYCT), New Jersey Transit (NJT), SEPTA, MBTA, and LACMTA have their own collection facilities and have trained urine collectors, STTs, and BATs on their staff. Most other employers contract out for these services, either directly or through a TPA or C/TPA. Specimens can be collected at a fixed location, at the employees' facilities, or at or near the employees' facilities using a collection vehicle. Either internal or contracted urine collectors, STTs, and BATs can be used at any of these locations.

The ideal environment for ensuring compliance with FTA **urine collection** requirements contains the following features:

- Clean rest rooms that are large enough to conduct an observed collection with sufficient personal space for the donor

- Sinks with electrical switches that allow the hot and cold running water to be turned off from outside of the rest room

- Absence of drop ceilings in the rest room

- A pressurized cold water system in the toilet tank that prevents access without dismantling the system

- Lockable storage containers suitable for securing valuables such as purses and wallets

However, these features cannot always be found in vendor fixed locations. They are found even less often at on-site employee facilities. On-site urine collection is often done in a typical rest room, shown in Figure 4-1, of a transit office building. These rest rooms are typically not secure. They may have places to hide clean urine specimens (e.g., above ceiling tiles) or may contain adulterants (hot and cold running water, soaps, cleaning chemicals).

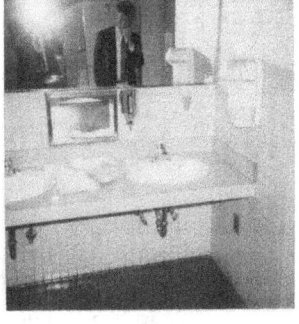

Figure 4-1. Typical Rest Room as Collection Site

One way to safeguard the process in an unsecured rest room is to have the collection technician stand inside the rest room but outside the private toilet stall (as shown in Figure 4-2) while the specimen is being produced. There are also several ways to secure the facilities.

One way to temporarily secure a water source at a sink is to install winged water faucet controls, drill holes in the holes in the wings, and put a metal bar between the wings. Another method is to place evidence tape over the faucet handles to prevent the donor from turning on the water or at least to enable the collector to detect tampering with the faucets. Evidence tape tears when someone tries to remove it. Masking tape, however, does not serve this purpose because it can be easily removed and reapplied.

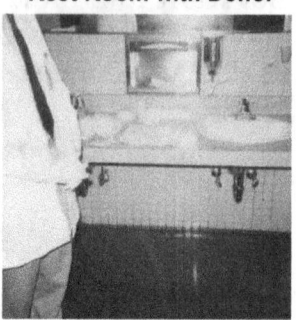

Figure 4-2. Collector in Rest Room with Donor

Evidence tape can also be placed across the tiles and frames of drop ceilings and on toilet tops to enable the collector to detect removal of fixtures. Waste baskets and toilet paper, paper towel, and Kleenex dispensers are common places for storing clean specimens and adulterants, and should be removed during the collection process.

Toilets and urinals with sensors, which cause automatic flushing when a person moves away from the fixture, should not be used because flushing washes out the bluing agent. Some collectors place masking tape over sensors with some success, though others have not found this approach useful.

Some collectors place tape over the flush handles to detect flushing of the colored water to get access to clear water. However, since the color of the water in the bowl would be clear, indicating the toilet had been flushed, the tape would only serve to detect replacement of bluing agent.

There are fewer concerns with **breath collection** facilities. Breath samples can be taken and analyzed in any room that is visually private and reasonably soundproofed, provided the equipment meets FTA specifications and is properly calibrated, the technician operating the equipment is properly trained, and precautions are taken to prevent contamination of breath samples.

Alcohol, alcohol swabs, and other contaminants should not be stored anywhere near breath collection and analysis equipment. One issue with the equipment is its height. It should be adjustable to make it easy for everyone to blow into.

HEIGHT OF BREATH COLLECTION EQUIPMENT

Metro-Dade Transit Agency (MDTA), a unionized system in Miami, Florida, experienced a grievance regarding placement of breath collection and analysis equipment on tables. Donors had difficulty blowing into the equipment when they were sitting down. In response, MDTA attached the collection and analysis equipment on a flat tray and mounted the tray on a jack. This assemblage was then placed on top of a chest of drawers. All of the necessary materials are kept in the drawers. The height of the collection and analysis device can be adjusted up or down to be at the same height as the mouth of the donor. The adjustable-height system is always level at any available height. The donors are now better able to provide a complete sample during the specified available time.

The bigger concern with breath testing is the cost and availability of the equipment. Evidential breath testing (EBT) devices are expensive and BATs have to be trained to use them. Many small operators are unable to afford EBT devices. EBT service agents are often difficult to find in rural areas. Many rural employers often arrange to use EBTs that are owned by other entities, e.g., trucking companies, school bus companies, railroads, small airstrips, U.S. Coast Guard. Most attempts to use EBTs owned by police departments have not proved successful.

Mobile collection facilities have become popular for both drug and alcohol testing. Many employers contract with mobile collection vendors, and some transit systems with large safety-sensitive work forces acquire vans, equip them with the necessary equipment, and hire full-time employees to staff them. For some operations, use of mobile facilities can reduce testing life-cycle costs. Merely driving the collection vehicles past employee facilities can have a deterrent effect. If properly configured and equipped, vehicles can provide a secure and comfortable environment for both urine and breath collection. Figures 4-3 through 4-8 show the mobile urine collection facility used by SuTran's vendor[2] in Sioux Falls, South Dakota.

The exterior of the collection vehicle, shown in Figures 4-3 and 4-4, looks like any other raised-roof van. It has a pair of side doors to provide access to the urine collection area. As

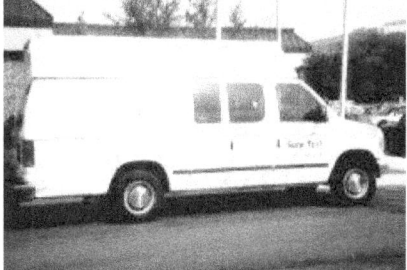

Figure 4-3. Side View of Collection Van

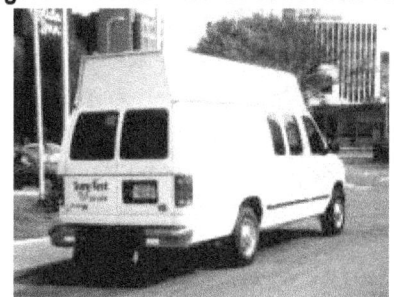

Figure 4- 4. Rear View of Collection Van

shown in Figure 4-5, a substantial step has been added to the rear bumper, to provide primary ingress/egress through the rear doors. The step should be designed so that it can be used safely in wet, icy, and snowy weather.

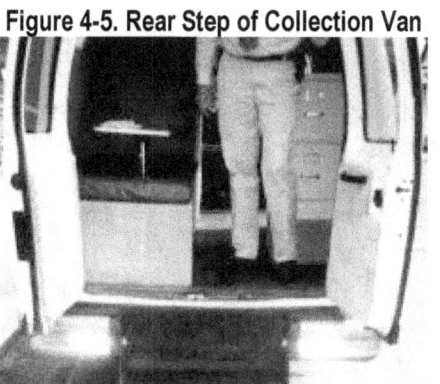

Figure 4-5. Rear Step of Collection Van

This van includes the required writing surface and benches adjacent to the rear doors, as shown in Figure 4-6. The space below the seats is used to store unopened urine collection kits, breath analysis equipment, and other materials.

---

2 Sure Test, Inc., P.O. Box 1840, Sioux Falls, SD 57101. FTA does not recommend or endorse Sure Test or any other company. The photos are included solely for reference purposes.

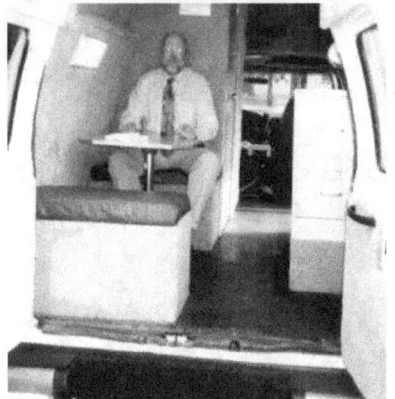

Figure 4-6. Interior of Collection Van

The two-drawer filing cabinet is used to store chain-of-custody forms, employer contact information, directions, and other printed information necessary to provide collection service. Interior walls are available for posting the collection procedures for the donor. Carpeting or other slip-resistant surface can be provided on the floor to maximize footing safety.

The space is reasonably comfortable for the collector and the donor to sit and complete all of the necessary forms. The gentleman in Figure 4-6 is approximately 6-feet tall and stocky.

Behind the collector is the enclosure that houses a standard recreational vehicle toilet, shown in Figure 4-7. The enclosure is large enough to allow a donor to produce a specimen without any discomfort, either standing or sitting. Between the enclosure and the operator's seat is the reservoir for water to fill the bowl and to eventually flush its contents.

A sink for hand washing, shown in Figure 4-8, is located behind the filing cabinet. The sink area

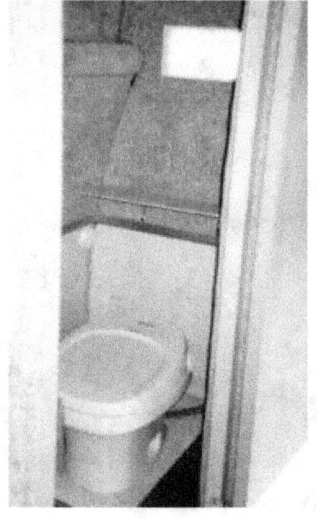

Figure 4-7. Toilet in Enclosure in Collection Van

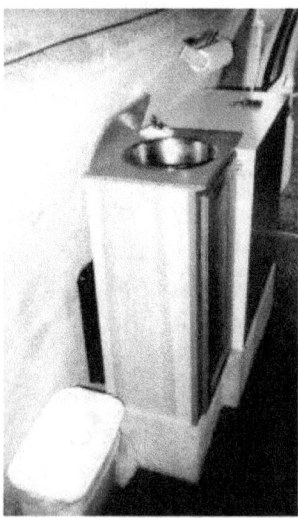

Figure 4-8. Sink in Collection Van

includes a towel rack for drying hands and a wastebasket for used towels and other materials.

Monitoring of Collection and Analysis Operations

To ensure compliant collection operations, employers should encourage feedback from and listen to employees who return from collection sites, and the program managers should regularly review the performance of all urine collection technicians, STTs, and BATs, whether they are internal staff, contracted service agents, or contractor or subrecipient staff. Program managers should talk to collection staff and ask them about their collection procedures and the type and amount of supervision of their performance.

Program managers should ensure that new collection technicians receive the initial training required in Part 40, and that all technicians receive the required refresher training. Development of standard forms and certificates can help in tracking and documenting the courses completed by the various technicians and the dates of completion. Program managers should also sample and evaluate data in the collection operation's central files. Reasons should be provided for all collections resulting in cancelled tests, either documented in the records or given during the review.

Common findings during audits of collection and analysis operations include EBT devices that are not calibrated, BATs who are not properly trained, and urine analysis laboratories with no recorded results for documented collections. Questions to ask during a review of a urine collection operation include:

- What precautions are taken to prevent clean samples from being placed in the collection room prior to a donor's arrival?

- How are observed collections handled when the donor and the collector are different genders (particularly when a collection vehicle is used to meet a donor at a remote location)?

- How often do "shy bladders" occur and how are they documented?

Questions to ask during a review of a breath collection and analysis operation include:

- What precautions are taken to prevent contamination of breath samples?

- How often do "shy lungs" occur and how are they documented?

- Has the EBT device been approved by the National Highway Traffic Safety Administration (NHTSA).

- How often does the manufacturer recommend calibrating the EBT device? (Ask to see the manufacturer's Quality Assurance Plan, QAP, for the device.)

- How often is the EBT device actually calibrated? (Ask to see the calibration log and compare it to the QAP.)

Mock collections should also be conducted at least once per year. Non-routine elements (e.g., a bottle of soap in a pocket for a urine collection or refusal to sign the form) should be included. In addition to noting any violations or errors or fatal flaws in the process, the evaluator should note whether the collections staff are aware of any errors or fatal flaws. A form used by Ohio DOT for documenting results of mock collections appears in Figure D-5.

It is also useful to schedule a few random tests (both drug and alcohol) during the 4 hours immediately after service ends, to ensure there is a facility for post-accident testing during that period.

Selection of Collection and Analysis Service Agents

The most common method of specimen collection is using a service agent's fixed location facility offering multiple services, such as occupational health practices or clinics, doctors' offices, hospitals, or testing laboratories. There are also specimen collection services that operate independently of any other medically related functions. These providers vary widely in terms of their business focus. There are also companies with specimen collection as their only business that fully understand FTA requirements for urine and/or breath collection. These companies are sometimes staffed with multiple trained technicians and/or medical doctors and can sometimes provide the level of service required. However, such companies are the exception. More often, the independent providers are secondary services provided by non-medical businesses. One audited specimen collection service was a small operation that was part of a computer software development company.

Entering an agreement with an FTA-compliant company with multiple offices in a spatially large service area that is open 24 hours a day and 7 days a week is often cost-effective for large and medium-size companies or consortia. However, such opportunities do not always exist. Alternatives include:

- Use of multiple fixed-location urine collection facilities for different times of the day, and for weekend days and holidays

- A collection service that comes to employees' facilities to collect a sample, using a standard rest room for urine collection and a private room for breath collection

- A collection service that uses a mobile collection facility

Use of a collection service with a mobile facility, for both drug and alcohol collection, is particularly common in rural areas among Section 5311 providers, where other services are not available at the times needed. Many other employers have found that the flexibility provided by collection vehicles significantly reduces system disruption costs. The vehicles can be deployed on any day, at any time, and to any location. Though the cost per collection is usually higher with a mobile collector than with a fixed-location collector, the life-cycle costs are often lower when service delays, supervisor time, additional vehicles, "deadhead" time, and transportation expenses are considered.

In addition to the practices discussed in Section 4.2 for selecting any service agent, evaluators should inquire about the training and supervision the urine collection technicians, STTs, and BATs receive and their procedures. The evaluators should also ask the questions suggested in the "Monitoring of Collection and Analysis Operations" discussion earlier in Section 4.3.

Perspective urine collectors should be asked to perform a detailed mock collection at their site for the evaluation panel. Perspective breath collectors should be asked to bring their screening devices and EBT devices to the interview and allow an evaluator to test them.

If emergency rooms propose to provide urine and/or breath collection, the collection staff should be asked how they will handle drug tests if all medical staff are involved with emergency treatment when a specimen donor arrives, and what they will do if a patient arrives with a severe emergency condition while a specimen collection is being performed.

A regularly updated list (once per month) of **urine analysis laboratories** that have been certified by the U.S. Department of Health and Human Services (DHHS) can be obtained from the Division of Workplace Programs, 5600 Fishers Lane, Rockwall II Building, Suite 815, Rockville, MD 20857, telephone: (301) 443-6014, or at http://www.health.org/workpl.htm. This list is also published in the Federal Register under the heading "Substance Abuse and Mental Health Services Administration (SAMHSA)."

Criteria for choosing between compliant laboratories are customer service, billing procedures, cost, reliability, and accuracy. Validity testing may influence cost. See FTA Drug and Alcohol Testing newsletters, particularly Bulletin 16.

4.4 Medical Review

This section discusses proven practices used by employers to manage the medical review process, to select MROs, and to monitor their performance.

Managing the Medical Review Process

Standard forms have proved useful in managing and documenting the various medical review functions. Examples of forms and lists used to assist with managing the medical review process appear in Appendix E.

The City of Albuquerque uses printed lists (shown in Figure E-1) to document and disseminate the roles and responsibilities of MROs. Albuquerque issues checklists to its MROs to guide them through the entire medical review process and to guide them in their interviews with tested employees (shown in Figures E-2 and E-3, respectively).

Use of standard forms provides records of various medical review occurrences, e.g., employee requests to test the split sample following a confirmed positive test result and an MRO's inability to contact a tested employee following a confirmed positive result. A split sample form issued by Ohio DOT to its subrecipients appears in Figure E-4. A failure to make contact form, prepared by University Services (Philadelphia, PA) for the Monroe County (Pennsylvania) Transportation Authority, appears in Figure E-5.

A flow chart of the verification process performed by an MRO (developed by the FTA drug and alcohol testing program audit team[3], based on the team's knowledge of the regulations and experience in evaluating grantees' medical review programs) appears in Figure E-6.

Selection of Medical Review Officers

Some large transit authorities, such as NYCT, NJT, SEPTA, MBTA, and LACMTA, hire MROs as employees. Most other employers contract out for MRO services, sometimes with companies that include support staff as well as several MROs, either directly or through a TPA or C/TPA. Prudent practices for selecting MROs are the same regardless of the administrative mechanism used to procure them.

There is no national registry of MROs. However, the American Association of Medical Review Officers (919-489-5407), the American Society of Addictive Medicine (301-656-3920), and the American College of Occupational and Environmental Medicine (847-228-6850) have many members who have the MRO qualifications required by FTA.

In addition to the practices discussed in Section 4.2 for selecting any service agent, employers should include the Part 40 qualification requirements in the procurement or solicitation device used to obtain medical review services or hire MROs as internal staff. Employers should also carefully examine the credentials of prospective MROs, and should meet with them and discuss their experience and knowledge about substance abuse disorders and their understanding of Parts 40 and 655 and how to interpret them. These discussions should include major medical review issues, such as how they handle prescription medications and over-the-counter (OTC) medications and what experience they have with donors claiming that herbal teas caused their positive test for marijuana.

---

[3] The FTA drug and alcohol testing program audits are performed by ICF Consulting and the Ketron Division of the Bionetics Corporation.

Monitoring Performance of Medical Review Officers

To ensure compliant collection operations, program managers should regularly review the performance of MROs, whether they are internal staff, contracted service agents, or contractor or subrecipient staff. All correspondence with MROs should be reviewed as it is received, to identify unusual situations that may indicate questionable performance. Data in the MRO office files should be sampled and evaluated regularly. Examples of unusual situations include long delays between test dates and reports of positive results that are later reversed, lack of timely response to communications, and errors on the type of test reported (i.e., pre-employment, reasonable suspicion, post-accident, random, return-to-duty, and follow-up).

One method used to monitor MRO performance is to maintain a matrix of tests by category and dates. Any pre-employment test dates occurring well after the hire date or well after any random tests suggest a categorization error. Multiple postings of the same test results suggest poor record maintenance and may suggest overall poor organizational management.

MRO reversals of positive tests reported by the laboratory should be questioned. There are a variety of legitimate reasons for reversing a positive, but legitimate cause for doing so occurs very infrequently. Reversal of more than a few positives per year for most companies is unusual, though some industries and locations have unusual circumstances. Nevertheless, such occurrences should be examined thoroughly.

Additionally, program managers should ensure that all MROs complete the continuing education units required by Part 40 within the required time frame. They should also establish a mechanism for receiving notification of all new hires of MROs, and review their qualifications to ensure compliance with Part 40. Development of standard forms and certificates will help in tracking and documenting the continuing education completed by MROs and in maintaining awareness of newly hired MROs and documenting their qualifications.

4.5 Records Management

As discussed in the *Implementation Guidelines*, drug and alcohol testing programs generate a large number of records that must be stored and maintained per Parts 40 and 655. These records are clearly designed to document that the required activities have been accomplished correctly. It is often useful to exceed FTA's retention requirements. It is particularly useful to maintain a contractor oversight file and to retain negative test result records for longer than the one year required. In fact, it may be in a system's best interest to retain all records indefinitely. This would provide useful data for scheduling random tests, and would provide a complete history of the overall testing program.

Record Keeping Methods

Part 655 does not specify how to organize records. However, a logical system is needed. Simple methods have worked best for many employers. There are two basic record keeping methods: (1) by test category and (2) by individual employee (by name or by identification number). The first method is used by many large authorities, e.g., Oahu Transit and Kauai Transit in Hawaii and the Transit Authority of River City (TARC) in Louisville, Kentucky. Use of a master log for each test category is helpful when using the test category method. The individual employee method can be very cumbersome unless the employer is small and has a stable work force. A third option is to file the information by date and by employee within each date file.

It is also useful to enter data from records into analysis files that can be used to evaluate the performance of the drug and alcohol testing program. For example, organizing the random test records so that the information can be easily collected and inserted into an Excel file to produce graphs will demonstrate whether the random tests were conducted across all hours of operation and across all service days.

Records Security and Access Control

To ensure compliance with FTA requirements for securing and controlling access to test records, employers should store all required records in locked filing cabinets in a locked room that can be entered only through a locked door. A combination lock should be used on the door to prevent unauthorized duplication of keys.

Records should not be kept in a room with drop ceilings with removable tiles. A person can remove the ceiling tiles in the hall in front of the records room, climb over the wall, and drop through the opening. A truly secure records room has wall partitions that abut and attach to the roof or ceiling of the building, thereby preventing anyone from climbing over the walls.

5. Referral, Evaluation, and Treatment

Employers with policies that call for automatic termination of any employee who violates the DOT/FTA drug and alcohol rules (i.e., a zero-tolerance policy) may want to devise a standard form listing the names, addresses, and telephone numbers of FTA-compliant substance abuse professionals (SAPs) in the local area. The form should also include the name of the violator, the date and nature of the violation, the date of effective termination, the date that the form was issued to the terminated employee, and the signature of the person who issues the form. Maintenance of such information would provide evidence of compliance with the referral requirements in Parts 40 and 655. In compiling the list of SAPs, these employers may also want to refer to the discussion of SAP selection later in this chapter (in Section 5.2).

Employers with second-chance policies, however, have much greater administrative responsibilities for referral, evaluation, and treatment of violators. This chapter discusses proven practices used by employers to manage this process, to select SAPs, and to monitor their performance.

5.1 Managing the Referral, Evaluation, and Treatment Process

Standard forms have proved useful in managing and documenting the various functions in this area. Examples of forms used to assist with managing the referral, evaluation, and treatment process appear in Appendix F.

To help employees better understand this process, employers with a second-chance policy may want to list the Part 40 requirements that pertain to the process and the role and responsibilities of SAPs, and to distribute the lists to all employees who violate the FTA drug and alcohol regulations.

To better ensure compliant return-to-duty and follow-up tests, many employers add the requirement that these tests be observed collections. This can be stipulated in the drug and alcohol policy, included in a list of requirements given to employees who enter treatment, or communicated to SAPs when they begin work for the employer.

Forms to document referrals provide records of employees referred to SAPs and the names and addresses of the SAPs. The City of Albuquerque uses a referral form (shown in Figure F-1) that informs the employee of the referral, lists the SAP referred to and an alternate SAP, designates the party responsible for payment, and requires a signature to acknowledge receipt of the referral. The Ohio Department of Transportation (DOT) uses the same form. The San Francisco Bay Area Rapid Transit (BART) District uses a form (shown in Figure

F-2) that includes documentation of the circumstances surrounding the referral and the SAP's findings and recommendations.

Many employers require employees to sign contracts, or agreements, documenting the conditions of their rehabilitation and continued employment. Ohio DOT issues agreement forms to its subrecipients to use when an employee enters treatment as a condition for continued employment and when the employee is approved for return to duty following successful completion of treatment. These forms appear in Figures F-3 and F-4, respectively.

The City of Albuquerque uses a form (shown in Figure F-5) to document all occurrences during the entire treatment and follow-up period, including the date and results of each rehabilitation test. This type of comprehensive form or a series of more specific forms documenting evaluations performed by SAPs and the treatment programs and tests that they order can be used as a case history summary of the SAP-client relationship. Such a summary can then be augmented with support documentation to complete the file.

The Massachusetts Bay Transportation Authority (MBTA) issues a standard evaluation form containing 28 "yes/no" questions (shown in Figure F-6) to SAPs. The SAPs are required to ask the questions to all new clients, record the answers on the form, apply prescribed point values to each answer (as shown in Figure F-6[4]), and tally the overall score. Another standard form, shown in Figure F-7, is used to document the specific requirements of the treatment plan devised for the client, who is required to sign the form. The form shown in Figure F-8 is used by the MBTA to document the SAP's evaluation of the client's performance during the treatment program, recommendations for further participation after the client returns to work, and the number of follow-up tests required of the client during the five years following return to duty.

San Francisco BART uses a follow-up assessment form (shown in Figure F-9) to document information regarding the treatment plan completed by a returning employee, the results of the evaluation following treatment, the date and results of the return-to-duty test, the SAP's recommendations for follow-up testing and treatment, and existence of a return to work contract.

Flow charts showing procedures used by the West Virginia DOT Division of Public Transit for return-to-duty testing and for follow-up testing appear in Figures F-10 and F-11, respectively.

---

[4] The instructions for the answer scoring and the scores appear in this example as sheet 3 of Figure F-6. The MBTA uses two separate forms for the questions and the scoring key, and repeats the questions on the scoring key form. The scoring key has been added to the form containing the questions in this example for convenience of presentation.

5.2 Selection of Substance Abuse Professionals

Some large transit authorities, such as the MBTA, hire SAPs as employees. Most employers, however, contract out for SAP services, either directly or through a TPA or C/TPA. Prudent practices for selecting SAPs are the same regardless of the administrative mechanism used to procure them.

There is no national registry of SAPs. However, the Substance Abuse Program Administration Association (800-672-7229) has many members who have the SAP qualifications required by FTA. Other employers have proved to be a good source for identifying local SAPs who have performed their duties well. Local SAPs are often most effective, since it is more convenient for them to meet face-to-face with their clients than it is for SAPs who are located a long distance from the employer's facilities. There are very few SAPs in rural areas.

In addition to the practices discussed in Section 4.2 for selecting any service agent, employers should include the FTA qualification requirements in the procurement or solicitation device used to contract with SAPs or hire them as internal staff. Employers should also carefully examine the credentials of prospective SAPs, ask them to submit sample forms they currently use in their practice, and meet with them and discuss their experience and knowledge about substance abuse disorders and their understanding of Parts 40 and 655 and how to interpret them. An important question to ask is whether they or the drug and alcohol program manager generates follow-up test programs. A number of audits have found that the employer devised the test schedule and imposed it on the SAP. A number of audits have also identified SAPs who do not understand their role as protector of public safety. Thus, prospective SAPs should be quizzed about their role. Another question to ask is how many tests are required of a rehabilitated employee during the first year of follow-up testing.

5.3 Monitoring Performance of Substance Abuse Professionals

To ensure compliant collection operations, program managers should regularly review the performance of SAPs, whether they are internal staff, contracted service agents, or contractor or subrecipient staff. All correspondence with SAPs should be reviewed as it is received, and all data in the SAP office files should be sampled and evaluated regularly, to ensure that the SAP monitors the clients throughout their treatment programs and to identify other questionable performance. One example of questionable performance is always prescribing six follow-up tests within a year of the client's return to duty. If this is done consistently for a large number of clients, the SAP may not be tailoring the testing program to the individual's needs. Another example is recommending a return-to-duty test soon after the employee tests positive on a random, reasonable suspicion, or post-accident test. The SAP may not have performed the required evaluations before recommending the test.

Additionally, program managers should ensure that all SAPs complete the continuing education units required by Part 40 within the required time frame. They should also establish a mechanism for receiving notification of all new hires of SAPs, and review their qualifications to ensure compliance with Part 40. Newly hired SAPs should also be asked the questioned suggested in Section 5.2. Development of standard forms and certificates will help in tracking and documenting the continuing education completed by SAPs and in maintaining awareness of newly hired SAPs and documenting their qualifications.

Appendix A. Example Policies

This appendix contains six compliant policies for entities that wish to develop their policy internally or oversee the work of consultants. Each of these examples is referenced and described in Chapter 2. The example policies are:

(1) Southwestern Ohio Regional Transit Authority/Cincinnati Metro

(2) Long Beach Transit (California)

(3) Tri-County Metropolitan Transit District/Tri-Met (Portland, Oregon)

(4) Des Moines Metropolitan Transit Authority (Iowa)

(5) Ohio Department of Transportation

(6) Georgia Department of Transportation

Each of these policies was audited and judged to be compliant with Part 40 before it was recently revised and with Parts 653 and 654, and each of them has been updated to address the revised Part 40 and Part 655. However, no policies have been audited for compliance with the revised Part 40 and Part 655.

The Cincinnati Metro and Long Beach Transit Policies included in this appendix have not been formally approved by their governing boards since they were revised.

---

1. Southwestern Ohio Regional Transit Authority/Cincinnati Metro

CINCINNATI METRO'S DRUG AND ALCOHOL PROGRAM--REV. 12/01

TABLE OF CONTENTS

PART I

CINCINNATI METRO'S DRUG & ALCOHOL PREVENTION PROGRAM

INTRODUCTION

The Metro is dedicated to providing safe, dependable, and economical transportation services to the Cincinnati and Hamilton County community. The Metro is also dedicated to providing a healthy, satisfying drug-and alcohol-free work environment for its employees. These obligations are severely jeopardized by an employee who is unfit for duty due to drug or alcohol usage.

Drugs and/or alcohol usage can cause work performance problems such as accidents, run delays, missing, and excessive absenteeism. It can cause sickness and workplace injuries resulting in higher health care and workers' compensation premiums. Drug and/or alcohol usage is also the cause of workplace accidents, damage to property and equipment, threats to public safety, including passengers and the general public and poor workplace decisions. Finally, drugs and/or alcohol usage can cause significant harm to the Metro's public image.

Drug and alcohol testing is mandated by the Federal Transit Administration (FTA) and the U.S Department of Transportation (DOT) in 49 CFR Part 40, and Part 655, as amended. In addition, drugs are prohibited in the workplace by the "The Drug-Free Workplace Act of 1988" located in 20 CFR Part 29.

Metro's Drug & Alcohol Prevention Program has been created to protect both the public and the Metro employees. It mandates discipline up to and including discharge, depending upon circumstances.. At the same time, it offers free substance abuse evaluation services and a second chance to employees who voluntarily come forward to the Metro and seek professional rehabilitation services prior to being notified of a pending drug or alcohol test. Metro's Drug and Alcohol program has been adopted by the SORTA Board of Trustees. This program is also intended to comply with all applicable federal regulations governing workplace anti-drug and alcohol abuse programs in the transit industry.

PART II

DRUG-FREE WORKPLACE ACT

SORTA/THE METRO
NOTICE TO EMPLOYEES

Pursuant to the
Drug-Free Workplace Act of 1988

The unlawful manufacture, distribution, dispensing, possession or use of all controlled substances is prohibited in SORTA/The Metro's workplace. Employees so found will be subject to discipline up to and including termination, depending upon circumstances.

Substance abuse is a major focus of today's society. The effect of this abuse on an employee's job performance is costly to the employee, his/her family and to the employer. In place is a testing procedure whose purpose is to insure a drug-free and alcohol-free workplace. No employee who unlawfully uses, is impaired by, or under the influence of, drugs and/or alcohol ever will be permitted to function in a position where his/her actions could affect the safe operation of a motor vehicle or endanger the safety of fellow workers.

Pamphlets on drug/alcohol abuse are available from the Nurse or Human Resources department. Also, SORTA/The Metro Employee Assistance Program is available to assist employees in receiving medical and rehabilitation treatment and counseling to help resolve substance abuse problems.

Employees found unlawfully using, impaired by, or under the influence of, controlled substance(s) and/or alcohol in the workplace will be immediately discharged. The employee may be referred to the Employee Assistance Program. Employees engaged in the unlawful manufacture, distribution, or dispensation, or found in possession, of an unprescribed controlled substance(s) and/or alcohol in the workplace will be subject to discipline up to and including termination, depending upon circumstances.

All employees must notify SORTA/The Metro of any criminal drug statute conviction for a violation occurring in the workplace no later than five days after any such conviction. Within 30 days, SORTA/The Metro will make a determination of action based on the incident. Employees will be subject to discipline up to and including termination, depending upon circumstances.

All employees are expected to abide by SORTA/The Metro's policy on a drug-free workplace.

PART III

CINCINNATI METRO'S DRUG & ALCOHOL TESTING POLICY

Bold Type = Required by FTA

1.0 APPLICABILITY

The Metro's policy applies to all employees. Certain portions, however, apply strictly to "safety-sensitive" employees (random testing) or "covered" employees (biennial testing, return-to-duty physical). "Covered" employees refer to applicants, bargaining unit personnel, Risk Management personnel, and any employees who drive or may drive Metro vehicles. **"Safety-sensitive" employees refer only to employees who perform job duties related to the safe operation of mass transit service including the operation, dispatch and control, maintenance, and supervisors who perform a safety-sensitive function and any employee who holds a Commercial Driver's License.** A list of "safety-sensitive" employee job titles is provided at Appendix A.

2.0 POLICY

The Metro is committed to a drug-free and alcohol-free workplace for the safety of its employees, its passengers and the public. That commitment is jeopardized every time an employee uses drugs or alcohol on the job, every time an employee reports to work with drugs or alcohol in his/her system, and every time an employee possesses, distributes, or sells unprescribed drugs.

It is the employee's responsibility to know and understand the Metro Drug & Alcohol Prevention Program. In undertaking this duty, the employee should pay close attention to Part IV, the consequences section, noting that termination may be a result of violation of the policy. The employee should also take advantage of the rehabilitation opportunities and awareness information available as explained in Part V.

This policy incorporates all of the requirements and procedures set forth by federal regulations 49 CFR part 40, 655, and the "Drug Free Workplace Act", as amended.

3.0 PROHIBITED SUBSTANCES

The presence of any prohibited substances in an employee's system is forbidden during working time. "Prohibited substances" addressed by this policy include the following:

3.1 Illegal Drugs

The use at any time of illegal substances identified in Schedules I through V of Section 202 of the Controlled Substance Act (21 U.S.C. 812), and as further defined by 21 CFR 1300.11 through 1300.15, is prohibited. This includes **Marijuana, Phencyclidine (PCP), Cocaine, Opiates, and Amphetamines,** as well as any drug not approved for medical use by the U.S. Drug Enforcement Administration of the U.S. Food and Drug Administration is prohibited.

3.2 Legal Drugs

The misuse or abuse of legal drugs is prohibited if it causes a positive test which cannot be medically explained and verified by the Medical Review Officer. All prescriptions must be administered properly, issued in the employee's name by a licensed doctor, and properly followed.

3.3 Alcohol

The use or ingestion of alcohol such that an employee has an alcohol concentration of 0.02 or above during working time **is prohibited.** (Refer to consequences section for the differences between a 0.02 and a 0.04). **Alcohol use means the consumption of any beverage, mixture, or preparation, including any medication containing alcohol.** The ingestion of alcohol up to four hours before the **performance of safety-sensitive functions is prohibited** regardless of the resulting alcohol concentration level. **The ingestion of alcohol for up to eight hours following an accident by any employee involved in the accident, as noted in part 5.5 of this policy, is prohibited unless the employee has already performed a post accident alcohol test in accordance with this policy.**

4.0 TESTING PROCEDURES

A prohibited substance may be detected through a drug or an alcohol test following the safeguards set forth by the Department of Transportation in 49 CFR Part 40, as amended. These safeguards are mandated to assure protection, integrity, validity, and the accuracy of the results. Discussion of collection procedures follows in Section 4.1.

Testing requirements call for urine tests for five drugs (Marijuana, PCP, Cocaine, Opiates, and Amphetamines) and breath tests for alcohol. This is subject to change consistent with alterations to 49 CFR Part 40, as amended. A separate test sample may be required for other prohibited substances based on individualized suspicion.

All testing will be conducted in a manner which assures a high degree of accuracy and reliability consistent with the Department of Transportation safeguards set forth in 49 CFR Part 40, as amended. Drug testing will be conducted in laboratories certified by the National Laboratory Certification Program as listed on the Substance Abuse and Mental Health Services Administration (SAMHSA), Department of Health and Human Services (HHS) notice located at 59 FR 39774 (see Appendix B for specific laboratory used by Metro). Collection may be observed if there is reason to believe that a particular individual may alter or substitute the specimen to be provided, as further described in 49 CFR part 40.25(e) (2) (i) – (iv).

Evidential Breath Testing (EBT) devices will meet the Model Specifications for Devices to Measure Breath Alcohol provided by the National Highway Traffic Safety Administration (NHTSA). Such EBTs will be listed on the NHTSA Conforming Products List publication found at 59 FR 18839.

4.1 Collection Process

The individual reporting to the test site must have some form of photographic identification to show to collection site personnel. If requested, the collector must show identification. The individual will be asked to remove unnecessary outer garments, such as coats and jackets, and to empty his or her pockets and display the items in them. Purses and briefcases remain with the outer garments, though wallets may be retained.

4.1.1 Drug Test Collection

The collector will have only one urine specimen collection under his/her supervision at one time. Unauthorized persons are not permitted in the designated collection area. The collection procedure is complete when the urine bottle has been sealed and initialed and the individual has departed the collection area or, in the case of an individual who cannot provide a complete specimen, the procedure is complete when the person has entered a waiting area.

The collector will be present during urine specimen collection. He or she will not observe the actual collection process (in cases where observation is not required). To the extent possible, a private stall will be provided for privacy reasons. Should use of a public restroom be required, no other persons will be permitted in the restroom, bluing agent will be placed in the commode if possible; a collector of the same gender will stay in the restroom but not in the stall of the restroom.

The individual will be asked to wash and dry his/her hands. After this is done, person must stay in the presence of the collector. The collector gives the person a sealed specimen bottle/cup and directs him/her to the lavatory. Nothing may be taken into the lavatory except the specimen bottle/cup. The individual will be told not to flush the commode.

When the specimen is returned, the collector inspects it for signs of adulteration and measures the specimen's temperature within four minutes of when the specimen was provided. A temperature in the range of 90 – 100 degrees F/32-38 degrees C is acceptable. If temperature is out of acceptable range, individual may have his/her oral temperature taken. This reading may provide evidence to counter the reason to believe the individual may have altered or substituted the specimen.

4.1.2 Urinalysis for Drugs

An initial screen will be conducted on each sample. If the initial screen is positive (as defined in Part III, Section 6), the sample will be tested again by a confirmatory Gas Chromatography/Mass Spectrometry (GC/MS) test.

4.1.3 Split Sample

The collector then divides the specimen into a 30ml primary specimen and a 15 ml split specimen (split sample). "Specimen A" bottle seal is placed over the 30ml bottle and the "Specimen B" seal is placed over the split sample bottle. The individual initials both seals. **If the sample also tests positive during the GC/MS, or is determined by the laboratory to be adulterated or substituted, and the MRO verifies the laboratory findings after review with the employee, the employee may request a test of the split-specimen. Such a request must be made in writing or verbally to the Medical Review Officer (MRO) within 72 hours of the time the MRO provides the notification to the employee that the test is verified positive, adulterated or substituted. The employee is not required to pay for the test from his or her own funds before the test takes place,** but Metro will seek reimbursement for the cost of the test.

The second laboratory is only required to run a confirmatory test for the specific substance which appeared in the primary sample. The results of this test must be immediately forwarded to the MRO. The MRO will notify the Metro and the employee of the result. **If the split sample reveals no measurable presence of the drug in question, the former positive test will be canceled** and the employee will be reimbursed for the split sample HHS laboratory test.

4.1.3.1 Completion of Drug Test Collection Process. The individual is asked to read and sign a statement on the appropriate "Federal Drug Testing Custody & Control Form" (Appendix C). This certifies that the specimen identified as having been collected from him/her is in fact the specimen he/she provided. All sections of the form are completed by the donor and the collector and the donor is given a copy of this form. The donor's participation is now complete.

The sealed specimens are placed in a secured refrigerator until pickup by the lab courier. The specimens are further sealed in a plastic pouch for transport to the testing lab.

4.1.4 Role of the Medical Review Officer (MRO)

An MRO is required to verify positive test results and facilitate the split sample process. An MRO is defined by the FTA as a licensed physician responsible for receiving laboratory results generated by an employer's drug testing program who has knowledge of substance abuse disorders. The MRO shall communicate all verified positive test results to the employee and to the Metro (see Appendix B for name and phone number of Metro's MRO). Upon the written consent of the employee, results received at the Metro will be forwarded to the President of the Union.

4.2 Alcohol Testing Process

Alcohol testing is performed by a Breath Alcohol Technician (BAT). An evidential breath testing (EBT)) machine is used to collect and analyze breath samples for any alcohol content. Results are read immediately. A screening test is given first; if results are greater than 0.02, a confirmation test is performed. One individual will be tested at a time and the BAT shall not leave the testing area. The procedure is as follows:

The BAT explains testing process and completes Step 1 on DOT Breath Alcohol Testing form (Appendix C). The individual completes Step 2 on form and signs the certification form. Note: Refusal to sign the certification is regarded as a refusal to take the test. The BAT opens an individually sealed mouthpiece in view of the person and attaches it to the EBT. The individual blows forcefully into the mouthpiece for at least six seconds or until the EBT gives the signal to stop. The BAT shows the results of the test. If results are less than 0.02, the BAT dates the testing form and signs the certification in Step 3. The individual signs and dates the form in Step 4. Testing is completed. Step 4 is completed by the employee only if the test result is 0.02 or higher.

If results are 0.02 or greater, a confirmation test must be performed. Prior to conducting the confirmation test, a waiting period of at least 15 minutes and not more than 30 minutes is observed. The BAT instructs the individual not to eat, drink or put any object or substance in his/her mouth and, to the extent possible, not belch during the waiting period. However, the test will be conducted even if these instructions are disregarded. A new mouthpiece is used for the confirmation test. Before confirmation testing begins, the BAT ensures that the EBT registers 0.00, if it does not register 0.00, testing must be done on another approved instrument. After the confirmation test is completed the individual is shown the readout of the results. NOTE: If confirmation results are 0.02 or greater, Metro is notified immediately. If the test result printed by the EBT does not match the displayed result or if a sequential test number printed by the EBT does not match the sequential test number displayed by the EBT prior to the confirmation test, the BAT shall note the disparity in the "Remarks" section of the testing form. Both the BAT and the individual shall initial and sign the notation. The test is considered invalid and the employee is so advised.

4.3 Return to Work Pending Test Results

An employee can return to work pending the drug test results under the following circumstances: Return to work physicals (when cause of leave is unrelated to drugs and/or alcohol and employee is not returning from inactive status), biennials, follow-up testing, and random testing.

An employee must await his/her negative test clearance under the following circumstances: return to work after a drug-and-alcohol-related leave, reasonable suspicion, post-accident testing, pre-employment and transfer to safety sensitive position or while an employee is in an inactive status.

NOTE: Employees are encouraged to schedule the return to work physical and screens in advance of the return date to avoid being in a non-pay status while awaiting clearance to return to work.

5.0 CAUSES FOR TESTING

Testing for drugs and alcohol will be conducted in the following circumstances:

5.1 Pre-Employment

All applicants are required to undergo pre-employment drug testing following the offer of employment. Employees are required to undergo drug & alcohol testing prior to transfer into a safety-sensitive position. Applicant screens will be offered with the pre-employment physical examination. If a pre-employment drug test is canceled, the covered employee or applicant is required to take another pre-employment drug test with a verified negative result.

5.2 Reasonable Suspicion

All employees are required to submit to drug and alcohol testing when at least one supervisor, manager or other company official who is trained in detecting the signs and symptoms of drug use and alcohol misuse reasonably questions the employee's fitness for duty. Reasonable suspicion will be based on specific, contemporaneous, articulable observations concerning the appearance, behavior, speech or body odors of the employee.

5.3 Return to Work/Return to Duty

Return to work drug and alcohol testing is required of all employees who have been absent for 30 days or more and are returning to hourly operations positions. **A return to duty test is required when a safety-sensitive employee or covered employee returns from a drug and/or alcohol treatment program as explained in Part V "Rehabilitation", or when the employer is made aware of an employee's treatment program.**

5.4 Follow-Up

A safety-sensitive or covered employee who returns to duty after a substance-related leave or after an evaluation made by a substance abuse professional is subject to unannounced follow-up testing. The frequency and duration of such testing will be solely determined by the substance abuse professional, but Metro will determine the actual days for follow-up testing. **The duration could extend up to 60 months with a minimum requirement of at least 6 tests within the first 12 month period.**

5.5 Post-Accident

This policy covers any accident involving either a revenue service vehicle, or a non-revenue service vehicle when the operator holds a Commercial Driver's License.

5.5.1 Fatality

Post-accident testing is required after accidents involving a fatality. As soon as possible, each surviving employee operating the mass transit vehicle at the time of the accident shall be tested.

An employee will also be tested if his or her performance could have contributed to the accident, as determined by a supervisor using the best information available at the time of the decision.

5.5.2 Bodily Injury or Property Damage

Post-accident testing is also required after an accident involving bodily injury requiring immediate medical attention away from the scene, or after an accident involving a vehicle which suffers disabling damage.

Such testing is required of all employees operating a vehicle at the time of the accident. As in the case of fatal accidents, other employees may be tested if a supervisor concludes, based on the best information available at the time, that the employee's performance could have contributed to the accident.

5.5.3 Reasonable Suspicion

Post-accident testing is always required after any accident that meets an FTA post accident threshold, if the supervisor reasonably believes that a driver's performance could have contributed to the accident.

5.5.4 Other Requirements

For post-accident testing, a urine specimen for drug testing must be collected as soon as possible but no later than 32 hours after the accident.

The alcohol test should be administered within two hours of the accident. If testing cannot be completed in two hours a report must be filed documenting why attempts were unsuccessful and attempts to collect must continue. If unable to obtain an alcohol test within 8 hours, attempts to collect must cease and the two hour written report is updated with an explanation as to the failure to collect.

The results of a urine test for the use of prohibited drugs, or the results of a breath test for the misuse of alcohol, conducted by Federal, State or local officials having independent authority for the test, shall be considered to meet the requirements of this section, provided such tests conform to the applicable Federal, State or local testing requirements, and that the test results are obtained by the employer. Such test results may be used only when the employer is unable to perform a post-accident test within the required period noted in paragraphs (a) and (b) of Section 655.44.

Except for the case of a fatality when the operator must be tested, a supervisor may decide, using the best information available at the time, that testing is unnecessary only when an employee's conduct can be completely discounted as a contributing factor to the accident.

5.6 Random

Random testing for drugs and alcohol will be performed on all employees filling safety-sensitive positions as listed in Appendix A which is hereby made a part of this program. Such random testing will be conducted at a minimum annual rate of 10% of the safety-sensitive workforce for alcohol and 50% for drugs, or at the rates set forth by the FTA in Part 655, as amended. Employees will be selected based on a computer-based random number generator that is matched with an employee name and identification number.

Random test dates are spread reasonably throughout the year (January – December) and are unannounced. Employees selected for random drug and/or alcohol testing are notified by a supervisor and must proceed immediately to the testing site with the supervisor.

Employees are on the clock and will be compensated at their applicable rate for the time spent in undergoing such random testing.

Metro shall provide to the Union, if requested, its scientifically-validated method of random selection for comment.

5.7 Biennial Physicals & Testing

An employee is required to take a drug and an alcohol test as part of his/her biennial fitness-for-duty examination (also referred to as the "biennial physical").

6.0 POSITIVE TEST

The Metro will be notified by the MRO of a verified positive drug test result. A verified positive test means a prohibited substance appearing in the employee's urine specimen which surpasses the thresholds established by the Department of Health and Human Services (HHS) as adopted by the Department of Transportation (DOT) in 49 CFR PART 40, as amended. These thresholds are determined by medical experts to be evidence that an illegal substance is in an employee's system (see Appendix D for threshold levels).

The Metro will be notified by the medical provider of an alcohol confirmation test result of 0.02 or more.

7.0 REFUSALS

An employee must follow the instruction and directions of all Metro supervisors and medical personnel involved in the testing process. A refusal means that an employee fails to provide a drug or alcohol testing sample as required by this policy without a valid medical explanation from a doctor chosen by the Metro, or engages in conduct that obstructs the testing process.

Refusals include, but are not limited to, the following: refusal to take the test, inability to provide sufficient quantities of breath or urine to be tested without a valid medical explanation from a doctor acceptable to the Metro, tampering with or attempting to adulterate the specimen or collection procedure, not reporting to the collection site in the time allotted, refusal to sign the testing form, or leaving the scene of an accident without a valid reason as determined by Metro before the tests have been conducted. A refusal constitutes a violation of Metro's policy.

Verbal or written refusal to provide a required breath specimen or to sign the DOT required testing form constitutes a refusal and is a violation of Metro's policy.

8.0 EVALUATIONS, REFERRALS, AND REHABILITATION

An employee concerned about his/her substance or alcohol usage should immediately seek assistance. Part V and Appendix E of this program discuss available resources.

9.0 TRAINING

All safety-sensitive employees are required to attend at least 60 minutes of training on the effects of prohibited drug use and the affects of alcohol misuse.

All managers responsible for covered employees are required to attend one hour of training for reasonable cause determinations for alcohol and one hour of reasonable cause determination training for drugs.

All employees attending such training will be required to sign an attendance sheet/certification form (see Appendix F).

10.0 SPECIMEN RETENTION

All negative urine specimens will be maintained by the laboratory for a period of one week. Positive specimens must be maintained by the laboratory in frozen storage for a period of one year (or longer if litigation is pending).

11.0 RECORDS RETENTION

The laboratory, unless otherwise instructed by the employer in writing, will maintain all records pertaining to a given urine specimen for a minimum of two years.

The MRO shall review or consider any medical information provided by the tested employee when a confirmed positive test could have resulted from legally prescribed medication. The medical information provided by the employee to the MRO as part of the testing verification may not be disclosed to any third party except in the case of a grievance, lawsuit or other proceeding initiated by or on behalf of the employee.

The employer shall maintain records of its anti-drug program for a minimum period as follows:

Five years: verified positive test results, documentations of refusals to test, covered employees referral to the Substance Abuse Professional (SAP) and copies of annual Management Information System (MIS) reports submitted to the FTA.

Two years: records related to the collection process and employee training.

One year: records of negative drug test results.

Such records shall be kept in a secured area with controlled access.

Records may be destroyed after 5 years at the discretion of the employer.

12.0 CONFIDENTIALITY

All test results are forwarded to the Personnel Manager in a sealed confidential envelope and will be kept confidential. In the case of positive drug or alcohol results, the MRO or BAT immediately notifies the Personnel Manager by phone so the employee may be immediately removed from performance of safety-sensitive duties. Test result information may only be released to the Employer, the employee, and to the President of the Union upon the employee's written consent. **In a grievance, hearing, lawsuit or other action involving the employee, the employer may release relevant information to the decision-maker, and to those who need to know the information to assist with the case. Such information may also be released to representatives from state or federal agencies when required.**

13 <u>CONTRACTORS</u>

Contractor organizations with persons who provide FTA-defined safety-sensitive functions for the Metro (including volunteers) will adopt an anti-drug and alcohol policy which complies with 49 CFR Part 655 and 40. No contractor employee who is in violation of this policy may work on Metro property or provide safety-sensitive services unless he or she has met return to work requirements (see Appendix G for contractor information).

14. <u>QUESTIONS</u>

Questions regarding any provisions of this policy should be directed to the Personnel Manager in the Human Resources Department (see Appendix B for contact name and phone number).

PART IV

CONSEQUENCES

NOTE: Circumstances not covered by policy will be dealt with on a case-by-case basis using a "reasonableness" standard.

The penalty for any violation of the "Substance Abuse Policy" or "Drug-Free Workplace Act" is discipline up to and including termination depending on circumstances. Violations include, but are not limited to the following:

1.0   Intoxication/Under the Influence

Reporting to work intoxicated/under the influence of alcohol or drugs (including all substances defined in the drug and alcohol testing policy on page 4) is absolutely forbidden. Any employee who reports to work intoxicated/under the influence will be terminated. An employee who is called into work unexpectedly has a responsibility to inform his/her supervisor immediately if he/she is unfit for duty. Otherwise, he/she will be treated the same as any other regularly scheduled or on-call employee.

2.0   Positive Test Result

Any employee who tests positive for drugs (as defined in Part III, Section 6.0) or has a breath alcohol concentration of 0.04 or more for alcohol at a biennial physical examination, return-to-work physical, post-accident test, reasonable suspicion test, random test, transfer to safety-sensitive position test or follow up testing will be terminated for the first offense.

3.0   Alcohol Concentration from 0.02 up to 0.0399

An employee who is on the clock, is tested and has an alcohol concentration of 0.02-0.0399 will be immediately removed from service and subject to a disciplinary suspension up to and including 30 days without pay (including sick pay). The employee will be required to sign a last chance agreement before returning to work. Repeat offenders will be discharged.

4.0   Refusal

Any employee who refuses to take a test (as defined in Part III, Section 7.0 of this Drug and Alcohol Program in the "Refusals" section) will be terminated. **Such a refusal constitutes a violation of Metro's policy.**

5.0   Manufacture, Trafficking, Possession and Use

The use, sale, manufacture, distribution or possession of drugs or alcohol while on the job, on Metro property, in a Metro uniform or while conducting transit authority business will be subject to discipline up to and including discharge, depending upon circumstances.

6.0   Criminal Drug Conviction at Workplace

Any employee who fails to notify the Metro of any criminal drug conviction or drug-related offense will be subject to discipline up to and including discharge, depending upon circumstances. This notification must be provided by the fifth day after such offense. Any employee convicted of such an offense will be subject to discipline up to and including discharge, depending upon circumstances.

7.0   Violation of Last Chance Agreement

Any employee who violates any term of a last chance agreement will be subject to discipline up to and including discharge, depending upon circumstances.

8.0   Alcohol Prohibited After Accident

Any safety sensitive employee required to take a post accident alcohol test is prohibited from alcohol use for eight hours following the accident or until the employee undergoes a post-accident alcohol test, whichever occurs first.

Any employee who is subject to post accident testing yet fails to remain readily available for such testing (including notifying employer representative of his or her location if he or she leaves the scene of the accident prior to submission to such test) is deemed to have refused to submit to testing and will be subject to discipline up to and including discharge, depending upon circumstances.

9.0   Alcohol Prohibited Before Workshift

Safety-sensitive employees are prohibited from consuming alcohol up to four hours before their workshift. Any employee found consuming alcohol within four hours of his/her workshift will be subject to discipline up to and including discharge, depending upon circumstances. (This does not imply that an employee's system will be free of alcohol after four hours of cessation).

10.0   Duty to Report

All Metro employees have a duty to report violations of this Program to the proper Metro officials. Any employee who has actual knowledge of a violation by any other Metro employee must report such violation. Failure to report is grounds for discipline up to and including discharge, depending upon circumstances.

11.0   Prescription/Over-the-Counter

Before beginning a work shift, an employee must report to his or her supervisor the use of prescription or over-the-counter drugs and other substances as described on page 4 of this drug and alcohol testing policy. It is the employee's responsibility to determine from the physician, practitioner, or pharmacist whether or not job performance would be impaired. A positive result whether illegal substances, illegal use of prescriptions, or misuse of prescriptions will result in discipline up to and including discharge, depending upon circumstances.

NOTE: There may be circumstances which arise that are not specifically covered by the above categories, yet, the severity of the offense warrants severe consequences. In these situations, the standard of "reasonableness" will apply and management shall determine the consequences based on this standard.

PART V

REHABILITATION

1.0   EMPLOYEE ASSISTANCE PROGRAM (EAP)

An Employee Assistance Program (EAP) is offered to Metro employees and their families at no cost to the employee. This program includes professionals qualified in the area of substance abuse evaluations and referrals.

The EAP offers counseling, evaluations, and referrals to rehabilitation programs. Counselors are available 24 hours a day (see Appendix B for EAP contact information).

2.0   SUBSTANCE ABUSE PROFESSIONAL (SAP)

Any safety-sensitive employee who tests positive for the presence of illegal drugs above the minimum thresholds set forth in 49 CFR Part 40 (see Appendix D), as amended, or who tests above 0.04 on an alcohol confirmation test will be subject to discipline up to and including discharge, depending upon circumstances. Even though discharged, the employee will be given a list of local and national resources specializing in the treatment of substance and alcohol abuse. Not all agencies may be qualified or willing to perform the duties of a Substance Abuse Professional (SAP). A Substance Abuse Professional (SAP) is a licensed or certified physician, psychologist, social worker, employee assistance professional, or addiction counselor (certified by one of the agencies in Part 40.281(a)(5) with knowledge of and clinical experience in the diagnosis and treatment of drug and/or alcohol-related disorders. Assessment by a SAP does not shield an employee from termination. (see Appendix B for contact name and information of Metro's SAP).

3.0   REHABILITATION

An employee who voluntarily comes forward to Metro (prior to notification of a pending drug/alcohol test) and seeks professional rehabilitation services for a substance abuse problem, either through the EAP or other bona fide treatment program, will be eligible for and required to sign a last-chance agreement. Any employee who signs a last-chance agreement cannot return to work until **he/she receives a written release from a Substance Abuse Professional stating he/she has properly followed the rehabilitation program prescribed by the Substance Abuse Professional.**

Under the last-chance agreement, the employee must complete a rehabilitation program and remain drug/alcohol-free thereafter. The employee will be required to sign a release of information form. **Follow up testing will be required after the employee returns to work. During this time, the employee is still subject to random testing.**

The Metro provides access to an Employee Assistance Program. All costs for rehabilitation services over and beyond Metro's EAP program shall be in accordance with the employee's benefit guidelines or at the employee's own expense.

4.0   CONFIDENTIALITY

Confidentiality of employees referred to the EAP will be maintained:

1. Employees must sign a release of information form authorizing EAP personnel and any involved treatment facility to advise Human Resources personnel on the progress of treatment.

2. Employees going through a substance abuse or alcohol detoxification program will be required to submit written documentation from the EAP as to the successful completion of the program.

Those who voluntarily seek treatment in an external treatment program outside the EAP must submit regular progress reports during treatment and a statement from the Substance Abuse Professional showing successful completion of the program.

5.0   LITERATURE

Drug and alcohol substance abuse prevention literature is available at a number of different sources. Through the Metro, employees can receive substance abuse literature from the occupational nurse, the EAP, and Human Resources. Additionally, material will be made available at the drug and alcohol prevention training courses as they occur.

Outside of the Metro, employees may access national or local hotlines and helplines, support group phone directories, treatment facilities, and many other resources for substance abuse information and guidance. Attached to this section is Appendix E which is a listing of agencies and telephone numbers available to Metro employees.

APPENDIX A: SAFETY-SENSITIVE

A.   "Safety-Sensitive" as defined by FTA 49 CFR 655:

Safety-sensitive function means any of the following duties:

(1)   Operating a revenue service vehicle, including when not in revenue service;

(2)   Operating a non-revenue service vehicle, when required to be operated by a holder of a Commercial Driver's License (CDL);

(3)   Controlling dispatch or movement of a revenue service vehicle;

(4)   Maintaining a revenue service vehicle or equipment used in revenue service;

(5)   Carrying a firearm for security purposes.

B. Metro's Safety-Sensitive Matrix

Gen. Repairperson	Claims Agent
P.M. Gen. Repairperson	Transportation Safety Specialist
Repairperson/Spotter	Industrial Safety Specialist
Gen. Serviceperson	Fare Systems Supervisor and Technician
Serviceperson	Supervisor of Scheduling and Control
Facilities service person	Maintenance Support Services - Manager
Gen. Facilities service person/Technician	Garage Managers
Repairperson (major shops)	Foremen
Electrician	Operators (FT & PT)
Unit Rebuilders/Transmission	Transit Traffic Controllers
Rebuilders/Engine	Board & Division Clerks
Unit Rebuilders/Electric	Government Square Supervisor
Repairperson – SR/CR	Government Square RCC Supervisor
Unit Rebuilders	Training Specialists
Machinist/Repairperson	Group Managers
Gen. Serviceperson (major shops)	Sector Managers
Repairperson/brakes/align	Division Directors
Repairperson/AC	Instructing Operators
Fuel Island Attendant	Line Instructors
Painter/Body Repairperson	Sub Clerks
Body Repairperson	Sub Supervisors
Body Repairperson/Trainee	Sub Dispatchers
Repairperson – CR	
Repairperson – Suspension	

APPENDIX B: CONTACT NAMES & NUMBERS

<u>Drug & Alcohol Program Manager</u>

Janice G. Smith
Personnel Manager
1014 Vine Street, 19th Floor
Cincinnati, Ohio 45202
(513) 632-7558 or ext. 558

<u>Drug Testing Laboratory</u>

Health Alliance Laboratory Services
Toxicology Lab
3200 Burnet Avenue
Cincinnati, Ohio 45229
(513) 585-6615

<u>Substance Abuse Professional (SAP)</u>

Dr. George Parsons
Associates for Psychological Services
Madison Road
Cincinnati, Ohio 45209
(513) 351-3334

<u>Medical Review Officer (MRO)</u>

Dr. Mary Jo Wakeman
OCCNET Health Alliance
3200 Burnet Avenue
Cincinnati, Ohio   45229
(513) 585-6488

or

Dr. Janet Cobb
OCCNET Health Alliance
2702 East Kemper Road
Cincinnati, Ohio   45241
(513) 771-223

APPENDIX C: FEDERAL TESTING FORMS

1. Sample DOT Drug Testing form

2. Sample Dot Breath Alcohol Testing form

APPENDIX D: DRUG SCREEN CUTOFF LEVELS

INITIAL CUTOFF LEVELS		CONFIRMATON CUTOFF LEVELS	
Marijuana Metabolites	50 ng/ml	Marijuana Metabolites	15 ng/ml
Cocaine Metabolites	300 ng/ml	Cocaine Metabolites	150 ng/ml
Opiate Metabolites	2000 ng/ml	Opiate Metabolites	2000 ng/ml
Phencyclidine	25 ng/ml	Phencyclidine	25 ng/ml
Amphetamines	1000 ng/ml	Amphetamines	500 ng/ml

Employees should note that thresholds are subject to change due to DOT requirements. Effort will be made to keep employees abreast of changes, however, it is the employee's responsibility to keep abreast of changes. Information regarding the thresholds may be obtained by reviewing the drug & alcohol regulations available at most public libraries or on the Internet at http://www.access.gpo.gov.

APPENDIX E: SUPPORT GROUPS AND OTHER RESOURCES

SUPPORT GROUPS AND OTHER RESOURCES

Alcoholics Anonymous	491-7181	Central Community Health Board	
		Drug Services	559-2056
		Children's Hospital	559-4200
AA Northern Kentucky	491-7181	Chaney Allen Center	556-4300
AAA Cincinnati Automobile Club	762-3111	Charlie's ¾ House	784-1853
Adult Children of Alcoholics,		Central Psychiatric Clinic	558-5823
AL-ANON, AL-ATTUNE	771-4070	Childrens Hospital	559-4200
Alcoholism Council	281-7880	Christ Hospital Alcohol/Drug Center	369-1116
Alcoholic Drop Inn Center	721-0643	Christ Hospital - Milestones (Outpatient)	421-7837
Alternatives (Talbert House residential		Cincinnati Union Bethel (CUB)	921-5838
treatment for adolescents)	761-9117	City Gospel Mission	241-5525/5526
Behavioral Counseling Services of Butler County Inc.	829-2121	Clermont Recovery Center	732-1710
Bethesda Alcohol & Drug Treatment Programs	489-6011	Comprehensive Care Center – Northern Kentucky Family Alcohol and Drug Counseling Services	(606) 431-2225
Bethesda Hospital	569-6014	Deaconess Recovery Center	861-6070
Bethesda Hospital Tel-Med	569-6231	CCHB-Drug Abuse Rehabilitation Enrichment Center	559-2053
Sample Tapes Available		Drug & Poison Information Center	558-5111
#942 Alcoholism		East Indiana Treatment Center	(812) 537-1668
#943 Is Drinking a Problem		Eighth Street House	291-8261/8262
#944 To Drink or Not to Drink		Emerson North Hospital	541-0135
#945 So You Love An Alcoholic		Family Services (Main Site)	381-6300
#946 How AA Can Help the Problem Drinker		Family Service of Northern Kentucky	291-1121
#136 Amphetamines and Barbiturates		Gateway Behavioral Health Network	861-4283
#137 Marijuana		Group Health Associates	872-2077
#138 Narcotics		Horizon Outpatient Program	
		Middletown	1-424-1193
		Hamilton County	851-2202
Brown Co. Counseling Service	1-378-4811	Ikron Institute	
		Industrial Counseling & Human	621-1118
		Resources Rehabilitation Center	621-1117
Brown & Adams Co.	1-378-	Intervention East	
Substance Abuse Center (Outpatient)	6068	(Seven Hills Neighborhood Services)	321-5329
Outpatient Care Unit Hospital	772-6969	Jewish Hospital (Adolescent Chemical Dependence Unit)	569-2015
Care Unit Hospital of Cincinnati	481-8822	Kenwood Psychological Services	984-3099
Center for Chemical Addictions Treatment (CCAT)	381-6672	Kids Helping Kids	575-7300
Center for Comprehensive Alcohol Treatment (CCAT)	381-6660	LifeWay Counseling Centers, Inc.	769-4600
		Margaret Mary Hospital (Batesville, IN)	(812) 934-6630

		NATIONAL HOTLINES AND HELP LINES	
Mental Health Services	321-8286		
East	471-6000		1-800-COCAINE
West	761-6222	800 Cocaine	
North central	541-7577	The American Council on Alcoholism Helpline	
Northwest		The National Council on Alcoholism And Drug Dependency Helpline	1-800-527-5344
			1-800-NCA-CALL
Norcen Behavioral Health Systems	761-6222	The National Institute on Drug Abuse Hotline	1-800-662-HELP
Northland Intervention Center	771-9112	Alcoholics Anonymous (A.A.)	212-686-1100
Prospect House	921-1613	Narcotics Anonymous (N.A.)	818-780-3951
Price Hill Clinic – LIFT	352-2538	Al-Anon	213-547-5800
Reading Youth Service Bureau	733-5623/4122		
Salvation Army	762-5600		
Sojourner Home	868-7654		
St. Elizabeth Medical Center Behavioral Health Center	578-5900		
St. Elizabeth North Adolescent & Adult	292-4148/4150		
St. Luke Alcohol & Drug Treatment Center	572-3500		
Substance Abusing Mentally Ill (SAMI)	281-6071		
Talbert House	751-7747		
Teen Challenge	221-2344		
Three Quarter House (Transitions)	491-4435		
Tough Love	232-0248		
Triple Outreach (Archdiocese of Cincinnati)	421-3131		
University Hospital	558-1000		
Psychiatric Emergency Service	558-8577		
Urban Appalachian Council	251-0202		
Urban Minority Alcohol and Drug Abuse Outreach	421-6005		
Program (UMADAOP)			
V.A. Medical Center	861-3100		
V.A. Drug & Alcohol Programs	559-5025/5027		
Volunteers of America	381-1954		
West End Health Center	621-2726		
Youth Counseling Program (Alcoholism Council)	281-7880		

APPENDIX F: TRAINING CERTIFICATION FORMS

1. Certification/sign in sheet for covered employees

2. Certification/sign in sheet for supervisory employees

APPENDIX G: CONTRACTOR INFORMATION

1. **First Group**
    Dennis Daugherty, Program Manager
    1801 Transpark Drive
    Cincinnati, Ohio 45229
    (513) 531-6888

2. **Firestone Mileage Sales Division**
    Anastasia Dreighton
    Human Resouce Representative
    17051 IH 35 North
    Schertz, TX   78154
    (210) 651-0214

2. Long Beach Transit Authority (California)

TABLE OF CONTENTS

Long Beach Transit Drug and Alcohol Policy

Bold = FTA requirements
Italics = Drug-Free Workplace Act of 1988 requirements

As an essential element of its commitment to provide safe and reliable transit service and to maintain a safe and healthy work environment for its employees, Long Beach Transit has had a drug and alcohol policy in force for a number of years, which has been strictly enforced.

The Federal Transit Administration (FTA) requires all transit systems to adopt a drug and alcohol policy that is almost identical with the existing policy of Long Beach Transit (the Company). While the policy of the Company applies to <u>all</u> employees, the FTA drug policy applies only to "safety-sensitive employees." It also gives additional grounds for the Company to test safety-sensitive employees. A list of safety-sensitive employees is included in Attachment 3.

Therefore, the existing drug and alcohol policy of the Company, as supplemented by the drug and alcohol program requirements of the FTA, is hereby adopted and confirmed as the Drug and Alcohol Policy of Long Beach Transit.

Illegal Drug Policy

The drug policy of the Company shall be as follows:

1. <u>Statement of Policy</u>

    The use of illegal drugs is prohibited.

2. <u>Application of Policy</u>

    This policy applies to all employees of Long Beach Transit.

3. <u>Definition of Illegal Drugs</u>

    An "illegal drug" is any drug which is not legally obtainable, or which is legally obtainable but has not been legally obtained, or is not being used for its prescribed purposes.

    No person should interpret any document, handbook, rule, statute, or regulation to be in conflict with the definition of illegal drugs or the meaning of the term "use" of drugs.

4. <u>The Use of an Illegal Drug(s) by an Employee is Prohibited and will Result in Termination</u>

    The use of any illegal drug or substance identified in Schedules I through V of Section 202 of the Controlled Substance Act (21 U.S.C. 812), as further defined by 21 CFR 1300.11 through 1300.15 is prohibited at all times unless a legal prescription has been written for the substance. This includes, but is not limited to, marijuana, amphetamines, opiates, phencyclidine (PCP), and cocaine, as well as any substance which causes the presence of these drugs or drug metabolites such as hemp-related products, coca leaves or any substance not approved for medical use by the U.S. Drug Enforcement Administration or the U.S. Food and Drug Administration. Illegal use includes use of any illegal drug, misuse of legally prescribed drugs, and use of illegally obtained prescription drugs.

The "use" of drugs means presence in the body system while you are on duty. A positive test is sufficient to support a finding of "use."

5. Testing for Illegal Drugs

When an employee does an unusual act, or has unusual behavior, which may suggest drug use, or has been off duty for an extended period of time, or has an attendance problem, or has an on-the-job injury, which requires medical attention, the employee will be tested. Applicants for employment will be tested before they are hired. All employees required to have a Commercial Driver's License (CDL) will also be tested whenever they undergo a physical examination for a Department of Motor Vehicles medical certificate.

6. Refusal to be Tested

A refusal to be tested will result in termination.

7. Positive Tests

If the initial drug screen is positive, a confirmation test of the urine sample will be conducted by an HHS-certified laboratory selected by Long Beach Transit. If the laboratory confirms the positive test, the employee will be terminated. It is not necessary that the employee be under the influence of the drug(s).

8. Disclosure of a Drug Problem

If an employee has a drug problem and voluntarily discloses it to the Company before a disciplinary matter develops and before being selected for testing, the Company will refer the employee to a substance abuse or chemical dependency program.

9. Prescriptions

When given a prescription by a physician, an employee must consult with his or her physician to make certain that the medicine will not affect the employee's ability to perform his or her duties and will not result in illegal drugs being in the body's system. When taking any prescribed medication that could affect the employee's job performance, the employee must notify the Company in advance.

10. Possession of Drugs

Consistent with the Drug-free Workplace Act of 1988, all employees are prohibited from engaging in the unlawful manufacture, distribution, dispensing, possession, or use of prohibited substances in the work place including Company premises, Company vehicles, while in uniform, or while on Company business.

In addition, all employees are required to notify the Drug and Alcohol Program Manager in the Human Resources Department of any criminal drug statute conviction for a violation occurring in the workplace within five days after such conviction.

Within 10 calendar days of receiving notice that an employee has been convicted of a criminal drug offense occurring in the workplace, the Company must provide written notice of the conviction to the FTA

Violations of these provisions will result in termination.

11. Application of FTA Drug Policy

The foregoing policy shall be in addition to the policy required by the FTA.

Drug Policy Required by the Federal Transit Administration (FTA)

12. FTA Policy

In addition to each of the foregoing provisions, Long Beach Transit shall also have the following drug policy **required by the FTA which shall be applicable only to safety-sensitive employees.**

13. Application of Policy

This policy shall apply to all employees who perform or are called upon to perform or may be called upon to perform a safety-sensitive function. Such employees shall be referred to as "safety-sensitive employees."

14. Definition of Safety-Sensitive Employees

A safety-sensitive employee is any employee whose duties relate to the safe operation of transportation services including: (a) operating a revenue vehicle, whether or not the vehicle is in service, (b) operating a non-revenue service vehicle, when required to be operated by a holder of a Commercial Driver's License (CDL); (c) controlling the dispatch or movement of a revenue service vehicle, (d) maintaining (including repairs, overhaul and rebuilding) a revenue service vehicle or equipment used in revenue service, (e) armed security personnel, or (f) supervisors who perform safety-sensitive duties.

15. Testing of Safety-Sensitive Employees

A safety-sensitive employee shall be tested for drugs as follows: (a) before an applicant or a non-safety-sensitive employee is allowed to per-form a safety-sensitive function for the first time; (b) after an accident; (c) when there is reasonable suspicion to believe a test is necessary; (e) on a random unannounced basis; and (f) for return-to-duty and follow-up purposes.

Safety-sensitive employees will be tested for marijuana, amphetamines, opiates, phencyclidine (PCP), and cocaine, as well as any substance which causes the presence of these drugs or drug metabolites, such as hemp-related products, coca leaves or any substance not approved for medical use by the U.S. Drug Enforcement Administration or the U.S. Food and Drug Administration. Illegal use includes the use of any illegal drug, misuse of legal prescribed drugs, and use of illegally obtained prescription drugs in accordance with DOT and FTA regulations.

16. Termination

A verified positive urine test shall result in termination. A refusal to be tested shall result in termination.

Alcohol Policy of Long Beach Transit or as Required by FTA

17. Use of Alcohol

The use of alcohol by any safety-sensitive employee, as defined in Sections 14 and 15 relating to drugs, is prohibited and will result in termination. **The "use" of alcohol by a safety-sensitive employee is defined as having an alcohol test result of 0.04 or greater while on duty, subject to duty, or just after performing a safety-sensitive function, as confirmed by an evidential breath testing device.**

18. Testing

The provisions of Section 5 and 15 relating to testing for drugs shall also apply to testing for alcohol.

19. Testing Results

Performing safety-sensitive duties with an alcohol concentration of 0.02 or greater is prohibited. A test result of less than 0.02, as evidenced by a breath-testing device shall be considered a "negative" test.

If the alcohol concentration is 0.02 or greater, as evidenced by a breath-testing device, a confirmation test will be performed. A confirmation test result equal to or greater than 0.02 but less than 0.04 will result in immediate removal of the employee from safety-sensitive functions for a period of eight hours or until a later re-test shows a concentration of less than 0.02.

A confirmed alcohol test of 0.04 or greater is a "positive test." A positive test will result in termination.

20. Refusal to be Tested for Alcohol

A refusal to be tested for alcohol will result in termination.

21. Possession of Alcohol

Consistent with the Drug-Free Workplace Act of 1988, the possession, purchase, sale, distribution, or consumption of alcohol while on duty, or while on Company premises, in a Company uniform, or in a Company vehicle is prohibited.

A violation of this provision will result in termination.

22. Alcohol Consumption

The Company prohibits the consumption of alcohol by an employee within eight hours before reporting for duty. **Any safety-sensitive employee involved in an accident must refrain from alcohol consumption for eight hours following the accident or until a post-accident alcohol test can be administered.**

Long Beach Transit/
FTA Drug and Alcohol Program Guidelines

I. Introduction

At Long Beach Transit, the safety of employees and customers is our number one priority. Both employees and customers have a right to expect a drug- and alcohol-free workplace. In 1991, the United States Congress passed the Omnibus Transportation Employee Testing Act, which requires drug and alcohol testing of safety-sensitive employees in the mass transit industry. In February 1994, the Department of Transportation published rules requiring agencies such as Long Beach Transit to implement specific drug and alcohol testing programs beginning January 1, 1995.

In response to these Federal requirements, and as a means of continuing our commitment to maintaining a safe and productive work environment, Long Beach Transit has revised its policies regarding drugs and alcohol to be in compliance with the Federal Transit Administration (FTA) rules on the Prevention of Prohibited Drug Use and Alcohol Misuse (49 CFR Part 655), and Procedures for Transportation Workplace Drug and Alcohol Testing Programs (49 CFR Part 40), as amended.

It is the goal of Long Beach Transit and the Amalgamated Transit Union Local 1589 to establish a work environment that is free of drugs and alcohol, and to foster a sober and drug-free work force. To achieve the drug-free environment that every transit rider, community member, and employee of Long Beach Transit is entitled to will require the best efforts of employees, management, and union leadership.

The following Guidelines have been developed as a help in administering Long Beach Transit's Drug and Alcohol Policy. As guidelines, they are not intended to be all-inclusive, nor are they intended to be used as hard fast rules regarding the application of the Company's Drug and Alcohol Policy in any particular case. Cases where substance abuse is at issue may be evaluated on the circumstances of that case and the Drug and Alcohol Policy applied as warranted by those circumstances. However, in those situations governed by regulations promulgated under federal authority, such as the U.S. Department of Transportation, **Federal Transit Administration**, or as required by state or local law, the applicable law will govern.

II. Contact Person

Questions regarding the Drug and Alcohol Policy or these guidelines should be referred to the Manager of Human Resources at (562) 591-8753.

III. Affected Employees

All Long Beach Transit employees are subject to the Drug and Alcohol Policy, including drug and alcohol testing. The only exceptions are the **random testing** and certain **alcohol provisions which apply only to safety-sensitive employees.**

IV. Definitions

For purposes of these Guidelines, the following definitions of terms apply. The definitions are written for explanatory purposes to help in working with this document.

Adulterated Specimen - A specimen that contains a substance that is not expected to be present in human urine, or contains a substance expected to be present but at a concentration so high that it is not consistent with human urine.

Alcohol Concentration - is expressed in terms of grams of alcohol per 210 liters of breath as measured by an evidential breath testing device.

Alcohol Use - The consumption of any beverage, mixture, or preparation, including medication, containing alcohol.

Canceled Test - a drug test that has been declared invalid by a Medical Review Officer. A canceled test is neither positive nor negative.

Chain of Custody - Procedures to account for the integrity of each urine specimen by tracking its handling and storage from point of specimen collection to final disposition.

Confirmation Test - In drug testing, a second analytical procedure to identify the presence of a specific drug or metabolite. In alcohol testing, a second test that provides quantitative data of alcohol concentration.

Dilute Specimen - A specimen with creatinine and specific gravity values that are lower than expected for human urine.

Employee Assistance Program (EAP) - A program provided by Long Beach Transit through Managed Health Network to assist employees and their families in dealing with drug or alcohol dependency and other personal problems. Assistance may be obtained confidentially by calling (800) 227-1060, 24 hours a day, seven days a week.

EBT - Evidential Breath Testing device used to measure breath alcohol concentration.

EMIT - An immunoassay test used as the initial drug screening technique to eliminate "negative" urine specimens from further testing.

FTA - Federal Transit Administration; an agency of the United States Department of Transportation.

GC/MS - A drug testing technique called the gas chromatography/mass spectrometry; used to confirm the presence of a specific drug or metabolite in the specimen.

Illegal Drugs - Any drug which is not legally obtainable, or which is legally obtainable but has not been legally obtained, or is not being used for its prescribed purpose or in the prescribed manner (this includes prescription drugs prescribed to someone else).

Invalid Test - The result of a drug test for a urine specimen that contains an unidentified adulterant or an unidentified substance, has the physical characteristics of or has an endogenous substance at abnormal concentration that prevents the laboratory from completing or obtaining a valid drug test result.

Legal Drugs - Legally obtained drugs (prescription and non-prescription remedies) used according to directions to alleviate a specific condition.

MRO (Medical Review Officer) - A licensed physician with knowledge of substance abuse disorders who is responsible for receiving laboratory results from drug tests; responsible for interpreting and evaluating an individual's confirmed positive test results together with his or her medical history and any other relevant biomedical information.

Metabolite - The specific substance produced when the human body metabolizes a given prohibited drug as it passes through the body and is excreted in urine.

Non-negative Test - A test result found to be adulterated, substitute, invalid, or positive for drug/drug metabolites. Non-negative results are considered a positive test or refusal to test if the MRO cannot determine legitimate medical explanation.

Positive Alcohol Test -The confirmed presence of alcohol in the body system at a concentration of 0.04 or greater as measured by an Evidential Breath Testing (EBT) device. Refusal to take a breath test without a valid medical explanation also constitutes a positive alcohol test.

Positive Drug Test - A confirmed test that shows the presence in the body system above the prescribed cut-off levels of a prohibited substance as verified by the MRO. A refusal to take a drug test without a valid medical explanation also constitutes a positive drug test.

Safety-Sensitive Employee - A safety-sensitive employee is any employee whose duties relate to the safe operation of transportation services including: (a) operating a revenue vehicle, whether or not the vehicle is in service, (b) operating a non-revenue service vehicle, when required to be operated by a holder of a Commercial Driver's License (CDL); (c) controlling the dispatch or movement of a revenue service vehicle, (d) maintaining (including repairs, overhaul and rebuilding) a revenue service vehicle or equipment used in revenue service, (e) armed security personnel, or (f) supervisors who perform safety-sensitive duties.

SAP (Substance Abuse Professional) - A licensed physician or a licensed and certified psychologist, social worker, employee assistance professional, or addiction counselor with knowledge of and clinical experience in the diagnosis and treatment of drug- and alcohol-related disorders.

Screening Test - Initial test. In drug testing, an immuno-assay screen to eliminate "negative" urine specimens from further analysis. In alcohol testing, an analytical procedure to determine whether an employee may have a prohibited concentration of alcohol in a breath specimen.

Substituted specimen - A specimen with creatinine and specific gravity values that are so diminished that they are not consistent with human urine.

Use - Presence of a prohibited substance in the body.

Validity Testing - The evaluation of the specimen to determine if it is consistent with normal human urine. The purpose of validity testing is to determine whether certain adulterants or foreign substances were added to the urine, if the urine was diluted, or if the specimen was substituted.

V. Employee Education and Training

Long Beach Transit believes that education and training of all employees in the effects and treatment of substance abuse will contribute to a safer and more efficient workplace for everyone. Therefore, educating and informing employees about the dangers of drug abuse or alcohol misuse and the possible penalties for violation of the Drug and Alcohol Policy are essential components of our program.

Safety–sensitive employees are required to undergo at least 60 minutes of training on the effects and consequences of drug use. All supervisors making reasonable suspicion determinations shall undergo 60 minutes of training in the detection of probable drug use and 60 minutes of training on alcohol misuse.

VI. Responsibilities

A. Employer

Long Beach Transit is responsible for developing and implementing substance abuse policies and programs that include drug and alcohol testing of employees and applicants for employment. The goals of these activities are to enhance productivity and safety for our employees and our customers, and to foster a sober and drug-free workforce.

B. Employee

Employees at all levels are responsible for reading, understanding, and adhering to the Long Beach Transit Drug and Alcohol Policy. This policy will be made available to all employees and the ATU, Local 1589.

C. Managers and Supervisors

Managers and supervisors will be held accountable for the consistent application and enforcement of the policy.

D. Union

Members of ATU, Local 1589, may have a Union representative present during any meeting related to a job action as a result of suspected or confirmed substance abuse policy violations.

VII. Enforcement

For any program to be effective, enforcement of policies is essential. Long Beach Transit will rigorously enforce its Drug and Alcohol Policy in order to protect the safety of our employees and customers, as well as to protect the efficiency of our operation.

It is the responsibility of all employees to ensure that the standards of performance contained in the Drug and Alcohol Policy are met. **Violations of the policy will result in removal from safety-sensitive duty** and discipline up to and including discharge.

A. Consequences for Policy Violation

1. Alcohol

Alcohol testing will be done by a National Highway Traffic Safety Administration (NHTSA) approved Evidential Breath Testing Device (EBT), which measures Breath Alcohol Concentration.

If a safety-sensitive employee's test result is equal to or greater than 0.02 but less than 0.04, the employee will immediately be removed from performing safety-sensitive duties for at least eight (8) hours or until another breath test is administered, and the result is less than 0.02.

Any safety-sensitive employee who has a test result equal to or greater than 0.02 but less than 0.04 on more than one occasion may be subject to discipline up to and including discharge. Employees will receive no pay for time lost as a result of a test result of 0.02 or greater.

If a safety-sensitive employee's confirmed alcohol test result is equal to or greater than 0.04, the employee will be removed from duty, and will be subject to discharge.

2. Ilegal Drugs

The presence of illegal drugs, as defined in the Policy section and Section IV of the guidelines, in the body system, while an employee is on duty is prohibited.

A positive urine test as defined by the current cut-off limits (see Attachment 4) is sufficient to support a finding of "use" for safety-sensitive employees for the following substances:

- Marijuana and metabolites
- Cocaine and metabolites
- Amphetamines and metabolites
- Opiates
- PCP (phencyclidine)

If test results are verified positive, the employee will be terminated. A positive dilute test result will be considered a positive test.

3. Refusal to be Tested

If an employee refuses to be tested, he or she will be subject to termination.

The following actions constitute a refusal to be tested by a safety-sensitive employee:

- Failure to appear for any test within a reasonable time, as determined by the Company, after being directed to do so by the Company.
- Failure to remain at the testing site until the testing process is complete;
- Failure to provide a urine or breath specimen for any drug or alcohol test required by DOT or FTA regulations;

- In the case of a directly observed or monitored collection in a drug test, failure to permit the observation or monitoring of your provision of a specimen;

- Failure to provide a sufficient amount of urine or breath when directed, and it has been determined, through a required medical evaluation, that there was no adequate medical explanation for the failure;

- Failure or decline to take a second test the Company or collector has directed you to take;

- Failure to undergo a medical examination or evaluation, as directed by the MRO as part of the verification process, or as directed by Long Beach Transit as part of the "shy bladder" procedures; or

- Failure to cooperate with any part of the testing process (e.g., refusal to empty pockets when so directed by the collector, behaving in a con-frontational way that disrupts the collection process) or verbal or written refusal to provide a required urine specimen.

- Failure to refrain from consuming alcohol within eight (8) hours following involvement in an accident without first having submitted to post accident/drug/alcohol tests.

- Failure to remain at the scene of an accident prior to submission to drug/alcohol tests without a legitimate explanation.

- Providing false information in connection with a drug test, or if verified to have falsified test results through adulteration, or substitution of a urine specimen.

- Failure or refusal to sign Step 2 of the Alcohol Testing Form.

B. Disputes

Long Beach Transit and Amalgamated Transit Union 1589 will work cooperatively to resolve issues relating to the application, and enforcement of the Drug and Alcohol Policy. Nothing in this program shall be interpreted so as to limit Long Beach Transit's right to assess disciplinary action, including termination, under the terms of the policy.

VIII. Circumstances Requiring Testing

A. Pre-Employment Testing

Drug and alcohol tests will be performed as part of the medical examination of all selected applicants. In order to be hired, an individual must pass drug and alcohol tests with a negative test result. Individuals who apply for positions at Long Beach Transit will be notified of this requirement at the time of application.

All applicants for safety-sensitive positions shall undergo urine drug testing and breath alcohol testing **prior to hire or transfer into a safety-sensitive position.**

All offers of employment for safety-sensitive positions shall be extended conditional upon the applicant passing a drug test and alcohol test. **An applicant shall not be hired into a safety-sensitive position unless the applicant takes a drug test with verified negative results,** and an alcohol concentration below 0.02.

A non-safety-sensitive employee shall not be placed, transferred or promoted into a covered position unless the employee takes a drug test with verified negative results and an alcohol concentration below 0.02.

If an applicant fails a pre-employment drug or alcohol test, the conditional offer of employment shall be rescinded

If an employee being placed, transferred, or promoted from a non-safety-sensitive position to a safety-sensitive position fails to pass a drug and/or alcohol test, they shall be subject to disciplinary action. (Refer to Section VII, Enforcement).

If a test is cancelled, the applicant/employee will be required to re-test with a negative test result. A negative dilute test result on a pre-employment test will require a re-test.

Applicants are required to report the name and contact information for all DOT covered employers for the previous two years. The applicant is required to provide a consent statement permitting the previous DOT covered employers to release drug and alcohol test results to the Company. Failure to provide information or provision of inaccurate or misleading information will result in immediate termination and/or rescission of employment offer. The outcome of the investigation may also result in termination and/or rescission of employment.

If more than 90 days have elapsed between the time of successfully completing pre-employment tests and the assignment of safety-sensitive duties, another pre-employment test will be required prior to the individual being assigned safety-sensitive duties.

Safety-sensitive employees who have been off duty for 90 days or more for any reason, and have been out of the random pool, must successfully pass a pre-employment drug test prior to the performance of a safety-sensitive function.

B. Reasonable Suspicion Testing

Employees are subject to reasonable suspicion testing. Reasonable suspicion testing is designed to provide a tool to identify employees who may pose a danger to themselves and others in the performance of their job duties.

Employees may be at work in a condition that raises concern regarding their safety or productivity. A supervisor must then make a decision as to whether reasonable suspicion exists to conclude that substance abuse may be causing the behavior.

A safety-sensitive employee may be required to submit to a drug and/or alcohol test, when a trained supervisor or manager reasonably suspects the employee has used a prohibited drug or has misused alcohol. The request to undergo a reasonable suspicion test will be based on specific, contemporaneous, articulable observations concerning the appearance, behavior, speech, or body odor of the employee.

Examples of reasonable suspicion include but are not limited to:

- Physical symptoms consistent with alcohol or drug abuse.
- Evidence of illegal alcohol or drug use, possession, sale, or delivery.
- Altercations (either physical or verbal) with others, or erratic or violent behavior.
- Other unusual acts or unusual behavior that may suggest drug or alcohol use.

C. Post-Accident Testing

1. Definition of Accident

Testing for prohibited drugs and alcohol will be conducted in the case of certain mass transit accidents. An accident as defined by the FTA is an occurrence associated with the operation of a vehicle in which:
- An individual dies, or
- An individual receives injuries requiring immediate transport to a medical treatment facility, or
- Any time one or more vehicles receive disabling damage. "Disabling damage" does not include damage to headlights, taillights, turn signals, horn, windshield wipers, and tires or other damage that could be remedied temporarily at the scene of the occurrence if special tools or parts were available.

This definition is not directed at vehicle collisions exclusively; it also includes incidents such as passenger or pedestrian injuries when the individual requires immediate transport to a medical treatment facility.

Testing for prohibited drugs and alcohol must be conducted when any of the above circumstances exist. The Company may send an employee for drug and alcohol testing following any accident, which does not meet the above thresholds if the supervisor makes a determination that a test is necessary.

2. Fatal Accident

Whenever there is a loss of human life, the surviving safety-sensitive employee operating the transit vehicle at the time of the accident must be tested. Safety-sensitive employees not on the vehicle (e.g., maintenance personnel) whose performance could have contributed to the accident (using the best information available at the time of the accident) must be tested.

3. Non-Fatal Accident

Following non-fatal accidents, the vehicle operator will be tested if one or more individuals receive injuries requiring immediate transport to a medical treatment facility or any time one or more vehicles receive disabling damage.

For non-fatal accidents, any other safety-sensitive employee whose performance could have contributed to the accident (as determined using the best information available at the time of the accident) will also be tested. However if an employee's performance can be completely discounted as a contributing factor, then he or she will not be tested under FTA.

4. Testing Guidelines

FTA post-accident drug and alcohol tests will be performed as soon as possible. Drug tests will be performed within 32 hours following the accident. Alcohol tests will be performed within 8 hours.

If an alcohol test is not administered within 2 hours following the accident, Long Beach Transit must document the reason the test was not performed and still attempt to administer the test. If an alcohol test is not administered within 8 hours following the accident, attempts to administer an alcohol test will be ended and a record will be filed explaining the circumstance surrounding the missed test.

The requirement to test for drugs and alcohol following an accident will in no way delay necessary medical attention for injured people or prohibit an employee from leaving the scene of an accident to obtain assistance in responding to the accident or to obtain necessary emergency medical care. However, the employee must remain readily available, which means that Long Beach Transit knows the location of the employee. Failure to remain readily available will be considered a refusal to test.

A safety-sensitive employee involved in an accident must refrain from alcohol consumption for eight (8) hours following the accident or until a post-accident alcohol test can be administered. A violation of this policy will result in termination.

When the Company is unable to perform a post-accident test in accordance with FTA regulations, it will use the results of Post-Accident drug and alcohol tests administered by State or local law enforcement personnel under their independent authority. This is acceptable only under limited circumstances, and the test results must be obtained in conformance with State and local law.

D. Random Testing

1. Requirement for Random Testing

FTA regulations require random testing of drugs and alcohol for all safety-sensitive employees. Random testing identifies employees who are using drugs or misusing alcohol but are able to use the predictability of other testing methods to escape detection. More importantly, it is widely believed that random testing serves as a strong deterrent against employees beginning or continuing prohibited drug use and misuse of alcohol.

2. Methodology for Random Testing

A scientifically valid random-number selection method to select safety-sensitive employees will be used. Long Beach Transit has purchased a computer program that will generate this selection. There is no discretion on the part of management or operations in the selection and notification of individuals for random testing.

The number of employees randomly selected for drug/alcohol testing during the calendar year shall be in accordance with FTA regulations. The current random testing rate for drugs established by FTA equals fifty percent of the number of covered employees in the pool and the random testing rate for alcohol established by FTA equals ten percent of the number of covered employees in the pool. A slightly higher percentage may be tested to provide for canceled tests. The test dates will be spread reasonably throughout the year. Every effort will be made to conduct testing on different days of the week and at different times throughout the annual cycle.

All safety-sensitive employees in the random pool will have an equal chance of being selected for testing and will remain in the pool, even after being tested. It is possible for some employees to be tested several times in one year, and other employees not to be tested for several years.

The process for testing will be unannounced and unpredictable as well as random. Once the employee has been notified that he or she has been selected for testing, he or she must then report immediately to the collection site.

E. Return-to-Duty and Follow-Up Testing

Under the Company's authority, an employee who voluntarily discloses a substance abuse problem, before a disciplinary matter develops and before being selected for a test, will be subject to return-to-duty and follow-up testing by the Company. The employee must be evaluated by a substance abuse professional, and pass a return-to-duty test. The purpose of this procedure is to provide some degree of assurance that the individual is presently free of alcohol and/or any prohibited drugs and is able to return to work without undue concern about continued substance abuse.

A return-to-duty test will include testing for both prohibited drugs and alcohol. The employee must have a negative drug test result and an alcohol test result of less than 0.02 to return to a safety-sensitive function. In addition, the employee must complete all return-to-duty requirements of the Company.

Once allowed to return to duty, an employee will be subject to unannounced follow-up testing for at least 12 but not more than 60 months. The frequency and duration of the follow-up testing will be recommended by a Substance Abuse Professional (refer to Section XII) with a minimum of six tests performed during the first twelve months after the employee has returned to duty.

Follow-up testing is separate from and in addition to the regular random testing program. Employees subject to follow-up testing will remain in the standard random pool and must be tested whenever their names come up for random testing.

IX. Drug Testing Procedures

It is not the intent of these guidelines to specify the requirements and protocol of the collection site personnel. These guidelines do, however, provide information about the requirements for employees and job applicants.

FTA-related testing procedures are as follows:

A. Drug Testing Methodology

1. Initial Test

Initial testing will be performed on the primary sample using the EMIT immunoassay technique. If the results are negative, no further testing will be required and a report will be provided to the MRO. The MRO is responsible for collecting, interpreting, and recording results and communicating results to Long Beach Transit.

2. Confirmation Test

Whenever a positive result is obtained on initial testing, confirmation testing will be automatically performed. This testing will also utilize the primary sample. All confirmations will be by quantitative analysis, i.e., Gas Chromatography/Mass Spectrometry (GC/MS). Results of confirmation testing will be immediately phoned to the MRO. If the test is positive, the secondary sample will be kept in frozen storage for one year from the date of its receipt to allow re-testing (see Section D below).

B. Applicant/Employee Drug Testing Requirements

1. Report to the specimen collection site as soon as possible after notification to report. Refusal to report for collection or refusal to cooperate with the collection process will result in a determination of a refusal to provide a specimen.

2. Picture identification must be presented, i.e. driver's license or employee ID. If identity cannot be verified, the collection will not proceed.

3. The individual will be required to check his or her belongings and remove any unnecessary outer garments, including purses, briefcases, bulky outerwear (sweaters, jackets, vests, etc The collector will request that the individual empty his or her pockets, display the items, and explain the need for them during the collection. The individual may retain his or her wallet. If any of the individual's items could be used as a potential adulterant, the collector may check it with the individual's other personal belongings.

4. The individual must rinse his or her hands with water and dry them.

5. Under normal circumstances collection site personnel will not observe the specimen collection. A specimen of at least 45 milliliters (about 1-½ ounces) of urine is required. The donor must urinate into the collection cup.

6. If the individual is unable to provide at least 45 ml, the collection site technician will instruct him or her to drink not more than 40 ounces of fluids during a period of up to three hours. The individual will then attempt to provide a complete sample using a fresh collection container. The original insufficient specimen will be discarded. If the individual is still unable to provide an adequate specimen, the insufficient specimen will be discarded, testing discontinued, and Long Beach Transit notified. The Medical Review Officer (MRO) will refer the individual for a

medical evaluation to determine whether the individual's inability to provide a specimen is genuine or constitutes refusal to submit to a drug test.

7. If the individual refuses to cooperate with the collection process, Long Beach Transit will be informed.

8. The specimen will be sealed and labeled in the presence of the donor. It then will be processed according to specific chain of custody procedures to account for the integrity of the specimen.

C. Observed Drug Collections

Procedures for collecting urine specimens shall allow individual privacy unless there is a reason to believe that a particular individual may alter or substitute the specimen to be provided. In the following circum-stances, the collection personnel must observe the second collection in compliance with FTA regulations:

1. The individual has presented a urine sample that falls outside the normal temperature range.

2. The collection site person observes conduct clearly and unequivocally indicating an attempt to substitute or adulterate the sample (e.g. substitutes urine in plain view, blue dye in specimen presented, etc.).

3. The laboratory reports to the MRO that a specimen is invalid, and the MRO reports to Long Beach Transit that there was not an adequate medical explanation for the result.

4. The MRO reports to Long Beach Transit that the original positive, adulterated, or substituted test result had to be cancelled because the test of the split specimen could not be performed.

Additionally, Long Beach Transit may authorize an observed collection when the test to be conducted is a return-to-duty or follow-up test.

The direct observation must be by a collection site person of the same gender as the employee being tested.

D. Drug Testing Split Sample

The urine specimen collected for FTA testing will be split and poured into two specimen bottles. This provides the employee or applicant with the option of having an analysis of the split sample performed at a second HHS laboratory should the primary specimen test result be verified positive. The employee or applicant has 72 hours after being informed by the MRO of a verified positive test to request a test of the split sample. All requests for split specimen analysis will be processed by the MRO, and sent to a second HHS laboratory.

Should the result of the second test be positive, Long Beach Transit will require the employee to reimburse the Company. Applicants are directly responsible for the cost of split sample testing under this provision, if they choose to exercise it.

X. Alcohol Testing

FTA regulations prohibit an employer from allowing an employee with an alcohol concentration of 0.04 or greater to perform any safety-sensitive duties. An employee with an alcohol concentration of 0.02 or greater but less than 0.04 must be removed from duty for eight (8) hours or until a re-test shows an alcohol concentration of less than 0.02.

An employee removed from work based on a violation of these conduct standards will not be paid for time missed.

A confirmed alcohol test of 0.04 or greater is a "positive test." A positive test will result in termination.

A. Alcohol Testing Methodology

A safety-sensitive employee may be tested just before, during, and following the performance of a safety-sensitive function, using an evidential breath-testing device (EBT).

B. Breath Alcohol Technician

Alcohol tests will be performed by a breath alcohol technician (BAT) who is trained to proficiency in the operation of the EBT being used and in the alcohol testing procedures specified in the Federal regulations.

C. Applicant/Employee Responsibilities

1. Present picture identification upon reporting for testing.

2. After testing procedures are explained, the employee and the BAT will complete, date, and sign the alcohol testing form. The form indicates that the employee is present and providing a breath specimen. The employee will receive a copy of the form.

3. An individually sealed, disposable mouth-piece will be given to the employee. The employee will be instructed to blow into the mouthpiece for at least six seconds or until an adequate amount of breath has been obtained. This initial test is considered a "screening test." The BAT will show the employee the result displayed on the EBT or the printed result.

4. If the result of the screening test is an alcohol concentration of less than 0.02, no further testing is required and the test will be reported to Long Beach Transit as a negative test. The employee may return to his or her safety-sensitive position.

5. If the result of the screening test is an alcohol concentration of 0.02 or greater, a confirmation test will be performed. The confirmation test will be conducted at least 15 minutes, but not more than 30 minutes, after the completion of the initial test. This delay prevents any accumulation of alcohol in the mouth from leading to an artificially high reading. The employee cannot eat, drink, or put any object

or substance in his or her mouth. The employee must not belch to the extent possible while awaiting the confirmation test.

6. If the initial and confirmatory test results are not identical, the confirmation test result is deemed to be the final result.

7. The BAT will sign and date the form. The employee will sign and date the certification statement, which includes a notice that the employee cannot perform safety-sensitive duties or operate a motor vehicle if the results are 0.02 or greater.

8. In the event an individual must be removed from safety-sensitive duties, the BAT will notify Long Beach Transit's representative immediately.

D. Incomplete Tests

If a screening or confirmatory test cannot be completed, the BAT must, if practicable, begin a new test using a new alcohol test form and a new sequential test number.

Refusal by an employee to complete and sign the alcohol testing form (at step 2), to provide breath, to provide an adequate amount of breath, or otherwise to cooperate with the collection process, will be noted on the form and the test will be terminated.

If an employee attempts and fails to provide an adequate amount of breath, the BAT must note this on the form and immediately contact Long Beach Transit. If no valid medical reason is determined, the inadequate amount of breath will be considered a refusal to test.

XI. Medical Review Officer

FTA drug testing laboratory results will be reviewed by a qualified Medical Review Officer (MRO). The purpose of this review is to verify and validate test results. The MRO is a licensed physician responsible for receiving laboratory results generated by Long Beach Transit's drug testing program. The MRO has knowledge of substance abuse disorders and has appropriate medical training to interpret and evaluate an individual's confirmed positive test result together with the individual's medical history and any other relevant biomedical information.

The MRO will perform various functions, including but not limited to the following:

1. Receive the results of drug tests.

2. Review and interpret an individual's confirmed non- negative test by a) reviewing the individual's medical history, including any medical records and biomedical information provided; b) affording the individual an opportunity to discuss the test results; and c) deciding whether there is a legitimate medical explanation for the result, including legally prescribed medication.

3. Notify each employee who has a verified positive test that the employee has 72 hours in which to request a test of the split specimen.

4. If, after the MRO makes all reasonable efforts, the MRO is unable to reach the individual directly, the MRO will contact the designated Long Beach Transit representative who will direct the individual to contact the MRO as soon as possible. If after making all reasonable efforts, the designated management official is unable to contact the employee, Long Beach Transit may place the employee on mandatory leave status.

5. Report each verified test result to the person designated by Long Beach Transit to receive results.

6. Maintain all necessary records and send test results to Long Beach Transit's drug and alcohol program manager.

7. Protect the employees' privacy and testing program confidentiality.

XII. Substance Abuse Professional (SAP)

A SAP is a professional who can determine what assistance, if any, an individual needs in resolving problems associated with prohibited drug use and/or alcohol misuse.

A safety-sensitive employee who has a verified positive drug and/or confirmed alcohol test result will be immediately removed from his or her safety-sensitive job duties. In addition, he or she will be advised of the resources available to evaluate and resolve problems associated with drug abuse, including the names, addresses, and telephone numbers of substance abuse professionals and counseling and treatment programs.

Referral to a SAP does not shield an employee from disciplinary action or guarantee employment or reinstatement with Long Beach Transit. Appropriate disciplinary action will be taken for all policy violations.

Employees may also be referred to a SAP after voluntarily disclosing a substance abuse problem.

XIII. Rehabilitation

Drug and alcohol abusers must be encouraged to make every effort to overcome the abuse and addiction that comes from use. Successful rehabilitation hinges upon users voluntarily rehabilitating themselves, with the assistance of outside professionals.

Employees of Long Beach Transit who have problems with drugs or alcohol misuse are strongly encouraged to seek help voluntarily. Long Beach Transit, through Managed Health Network, provides an Employee Assistance Program (EAP) to assist employees in dealing with drug- and alcohol-related problems. The EAP is one means for rehabilitation and can be contacted at (800) 227-1060 24 hours a day, 7 days a week. In addition, all employees are encouraged to make use of other available resources for treatment of substance abuse problems.

Voluntary enrollment in a rehabilitation program does not excuse or exempt an employee from discipline if he or she tests positive for drugs while on duty or for alcohol just before, during, or following the performance of a safety-sensitive function.

XIV. Confidentiality

Laboratory reports or test results for FTA testing will not appear in a safety-sensitive employee's personnel file. Information of this nature, however, will be included in a separate confidential medical folder maintained in a confidential manner. The reports or test results may be disclosed to Long Beach Transit management on a strictly need-to-know basis and to the tested employee upon request by a written signed release. Disclosure, without employee consent, may also occur when:

- The disclosure is compelled by legal proceedings, (civil or criminal). These proceedings include a lawsuit (e.g., a wrongful discharge action), grievance (e.g., an arbitration concerning disciplinary action taken by the employer), or administrative proceeding (e.g., an unemployment compensation hearing) brought by, or on behalf of, an employee and resulting from a positive DOT drug or alcohol test or a refusal to test (including, but not limited to, adulterated, or substituted test results). These proceedings also include a criminal or civil action resulting from an employee's performance of safety-sensitive duties. In such a proceeding, the release of information to the decision maker in the proceeding (e.g., the court in a lawsuit) will only be released with a binding stipulation that the decision maker to whom it is released will make it available only to parties to the proceeding.

- The information is requested by the DOT, FTA or any DOT agency, or federal, state, or local safety agency with regulatory authority over Long Beach Transit or any of its employees.

- The information is requested by a subsequent employer (if the employee has expressly authorized the particular records be transmitted to that employer);

- The information has been placed at issue in a formal dispute between the tested employee or applicant and Long Beach Transit;

- The information is needed by medical personnel for the diagnosis or treatment of the employee or applicant who is unable to authorize disclosure;

- The information is requested by the National Transportation Safety Board during an accident investigation; or

- In cases of a contractor or sub-recipient of a state department of transportation, records will be released when requested by such agencies that must certify compliance with the regulation to the FTA.

XV. Effective Date

The effective date of these revised guidelines is February 2002.

Attachment 1

Drug and Alcohol Abuse Information Helplines

Mona Gillman
Substance Abuse Professional
(714) 567-4845

Managed Health Network (EAP)
(800) 227-1060

Alcohol and Drug Referral Hotline
(800) 252-6465

American Council on Alcoholism Hot Line
(800) 356-9996

Al-Anon
(800) 344-2666

Center for Substance Abuse Treatment
(800) 662-4357

Mothers Against Drunk Driving (MADD)
(800) 438-6233

National Cocaine Hot Line
(800) 262-2463

National Institute on Drug Abuse Hot Line
(800) 662-HELP

Attachment 2

Health and Safety Issues
Related to Drug Abuse and Alcohol Misuse

Substance abuse, the misuse of drugs and alcohol, is not a new issue, but it is one of growing concern to employers. Substance abuse is a problem in the workplace. Research has shown that substance abuse affects organizations, as evidenced by increased medical benefit claims, increased absenteeism, increased worker's compensation claims, and decreased productivity. Substance abuse poses serious safety and health risks not only to the user, but also to those who work with or come into contact with the user. As a result, employers have become even more concerned about the misuse of drugs and alcohol by employees who perform safety-sensitive functions in the organization, and in functions involving direct contact with the public.

Alcohol Facts

Alcohol, when consumed primarily for its physical and mood-altering effects, is a substance of abuse. As a depressant it slows down physical responses and progressively impairs mental functions. Signs and symptoms of use include dulled mental processes, lack of coordination, odor of alcohol on the breath, slowed reaction rate, and slurred speech. The chronic consumption of alcohol over time may result in decreased sexual functioning, dependency, fatal liver disease, kidney disease, and birth defects.

It takes one hour for the average person (150 pounds) to process one serving of an alcoholic beverage from the body. Impairment in coordination and judgement can be objectively measured with as little as two drinks in the body. A person who is legally intoxicated is six times more likely to have an accident than a sober person.

Amphetamine Facts

Amphetamines are central nervous system stimulants that speed up the mind and body. Signs and symptoms of use include hyperexcitability, restlessness, confusion, panic, talkativeness, inability to concentrate, and heightened aggressive behavior. Regular use produces strong psychological dependence and increasing tolerance to the drug.

Low-dose amphetamine use will cause short-term improvement in mental and physical functioning. With greater use, however, the effect reverses and has an impairing effect. Hangover effect is characterized by physical fatigue and depression, which may make operation of equipment or vehicles dangerous.

Cocaine Facts

Cocaine is abused as a powerful physical and mental stimulant; the entire central nervous system is energized. Signs and symptoms of use include financial problems, increased physical activity and fatigue, isolation and withdrawal from friends and normal activities, unusual defensiveness, anxiety, agitation, and wide mood swings. Cocaine use causes the heart to beat faster and harder and rapidly increases blood pressure. Cocaine causes spasms of blood vessels in the brain and heart and can lead to ruptured vessels causing strokes or heart attacks. Extreme mood and energy swings create instability. Work performance is characterized by forgetfulness, absenteeism, tardiness, and missed assignments.

Marijuana Facts

People use marijuana for the mildly tranquilizing, mood altering and perception altering effects it produces. Signs and symptoms of use include reddened eyes, slowed speech, chronic fatigue, and lack of motivation. Chronic smoking of marijuana causes emphysema-like conditions. Regular use can cause diminished concentration, impaired short-term memory, impaired signal detection, and impaired tracking (the ability to follow a moving object with the eye).

Marijuana smoking has a long-term effect on performance. Combining alcohol and other depressant drugs and marijuana can produce a multiplied effect, increasing the impairing effect of both the depressant and marijuana.

Opiates (Narcotics) Facts

Opiates (also called narcotics) are drugs that alleviate pain, depress body functions, and when taken in large doses, cause a strong euphoric feeling. Signs and symptoms of use include mood changes, impaired mental functioning, depression and apathy, impaired coordination, and physical fatigue and drowsiness. IV needle users have a high risk for contracting hepatitis and AIDS due to sharing of needles.

Unwanted side effects of opiates such as nausea, vomiting, dizziness, mental clouding, and drowsiness place the legitimate user and abuser at higher risk for an accident. Workplace use may cause impairment of physical and mental functions.

Phencyclidine (PCP) Facts

Phencyclidine acts as both a depressant and a hallucinogen, and sometimes a stimulant. Signs and symptoms of use include impaired coordination, severe confusion and agitation, extreme mood shifts, rapid heartbeat, and dizziness. The potential for accidents and overdose is high due to the extreme mental effects combined with the anesthetic effect on the body. PCP use can cause irreversible memory loss, personality changes, and thought disorders.

Attachment 3

List of Safety-Sensitive Employees

- Motor Coach Operator

- Student Operator

- Operations Supervisor

- Operations Lead Supervisor

- Maintenance Supervisor

- "A" Mechanic

- "B" Mechanic

- "C" Mechanic

- Utility Worker

- Training Supervisors

- Lead Training Supervisor

- Safety Officer

Attachment 4

Minimum Thresholds

INITIAL TEST CUT-OFF LEVELS

	(ng/ml)
Marijuana metabolites	50
Cocaine metabolites	300
Opiate metabolites	2,000
Phencyclidine	25
Amphetamines	1,000

CONFIRMATORY TEST CUT-OFF LEVELS

	(ng/ml)
Marijuana metabolites	15
Cocaine metabolites	150
Opiates:	
Morphine	2,000
Codeine	2,000
Phencyclidine	25
Amphetamines:	
Amphetamines	500
Methamphetamine	500

Delta-9-tetrahydrocannabinol-9-carboxylic acid.
Benzoylecgonine
Specimen must also contain amphetamine at a concentration greater than or equal to 200 ng/ml.

Attachment 5

List of Contacts

Any questions regarding this policy or any other aspect of the substance abuse policy should be directed to the following individual(s).

Drug and Alcohol Program Manager

Name:	LaVerne David
Title:	Manager, Human Resources
Address:	Long Beach Transit
Telephone No:	(562) 591-8753

Drug and Alcohol Program Administrator

Name:	Jacqueline Gomez
Title:	Human Resources Assistant
Address:	Long Beach Transit
Telephone No:	(562) 591-8753

Medical Review Officer

Name:	Drs. Brian and Helen Tang
Title:	Medical Review Officers
Address:	Long Beach Medical Clinic
Telephone No:	(562) 437-0831

Substance Abuse Professional

Name:	Mona Gillman
Title:	Substance Abuse Professional
Address:	Long Beach, CA
Telephone No:	(714) 567-4845

HHS Certified Laboratory

Name:	Pacific Toxicology Laboratories
Address:	Woodland Hills, CA
Telephone No:	(818) 598-3110

3. Tri-County Metropolitan Transit District/Tri-Met (Portland, Oregon)

TABLE OF CONTENTS

TRI-MET
DRUG AND ALCOHOL ABUSE POLICY

Effective March 27, 2002

A. INTRODUCTION

The District has the responsibility to its customers and the general public to provide safe, efficient transportation services while insuring safe working conditions for its employees. To satisfy these responsibilities, the District must establish a work environment where its employees are free from the effects of drugs or alcohol.

B. APPLICABILITY

This Policy applies to all District employees and certain contracted employees.

C. PURPOSE

The purpose of this Policy is to assure employee fitness for duty and to protect District employees, customers, and the public from risk posed by worker use of drugs or alcohol. This Policy is intended to comply with all applicable Federal regulations governing workplace drug use and alcohol misuse in the transit industry. Regulations issued by the U.S. Department of Transportation (DOT) and the Federal Transit Administration (FTA) mandate urine drug testing and evidential breath alcohol testing for safety-sensitive positions. This Policy sets forth the District drug and alcohol abuse program and the testing and reporting guidelines for safety-sensitive employees as required by those regulations, and for employees in non-safety-sensitive positions.

It is the goal of this Policy to prevent substance abuse and rehabilitate rather than terminate the employment of workers. However, all persons covered by this Policy should be aware that violations of the Policy will result in discipline, up to and including termination, or in not being hired.

Compliance with DOT/FTA drug and alcohol regulations and District policy is a condition of employment.

D. PROHIBITED SUBSTANCES

The FTA Regulations prohibit the consumption of the following drugs and drug metabolites at any time: marijuana, amphetamines, opiates, phencyclidine (PCP), and cocaine. In addition to the aforementioned drugs, it is the District's policy to prohibit any illegal controlled substance, as well as any drug not approved for medical use by the USDA or the USFDA. Illegal use includes use of, or impairment by, any illegal drug, misuse of legally prescribed or over-the-counter drugs, or illegally obtained prescription drugs.

With respect to safety-sensitive employees, the FTA prohibits the consumption of any alcoholic substance, beverage, or mixture, including any medication containing alcohol within four (4) hours of the employee's scheduled time to report for work, while on duty or within eight (8) hours following an accident or until the employee takes a post-accident alcohol and/or drug test, whichever occurs first.

Under District policy, the aforementioned prohibition applies to all employees.

E. PROHIBITED BEHAVIOR

The use, possession, distribution, sale, purchase, manufacture, dispensation of or intoxication by alcoholic substances or beverages, intoxicants, illegal drugs, controlled substances not medically authorized, related drug paraphernalia, or other substances including prescription drugs which impair job performance or mental or motor function by any employee or any other person to whom this Policy applies while on District premises or in the course of conducting District business during regular business hours, including while subject to being on-call in a paid status, at lunch or on breaks, is strictly prohibited. Safety-sensitive employees are prohibited from the consumption of illegal drugs at all times.

Employees performing safety-sensitive job functions are prohibited from reporting to or remaining on duty with an alcohol concentration level of 0.02 or greater. Safety-sensitive employees may not use alcohol from any source while on duty or within four (4) hours prior to performing safety-sensitive duty.

Safety-sensitive employees on call are prohibited from using alcohol during hours they are on on-call paid status. Any time an employee (not on paid status) is called to report for duty, and the employee has used alcohol within 4 hours of the call, the employee must turn down the work or acknowledge the use of alcohol and the inability to perform the safety-sensitive function.

Employees who are reasonably suspected of engaging in a prohibited activity, or of not being fit for duty due to drug or alcohol misuse will be suspended from duty pending an investigation and verification. Employees who fail to pass a drug or alcohol test, or who engage in a prohibited activity will be removed from duty and subject to disciplinary action, up to and including discharge.

F. ALCOHOL

1. ADVERSE EFFECTS

It is recognized that alcohol is a legal, socially acceptable drug when consumed in moderation. However, when consumed primarily for its physical and mood-altering effects, it is a substance that is subject to abuse. As a depressant, it slows physical responses and progressively impairs mental functions, including the ability to safely operate a motorized vehicle or machinery. The chronic consumption of alcohol over time may result in critical health issues, including dependency, fatal liver diseases, ulcers, and increased possibility of cancers. Slurred speech, poor coordination, inability to walk straight, rapid eye movement, impaired attention or memory, stupor or coma are all signs of alcohol use and problems.

If an alcohol problem is suspected the Employee Assistance Program and/or the Drug and Alcohol Coordinator should be contacted.

2. USE

The FTA requires that no safety-sensitive employee shall report for duty within four (4) hours of using any alcoholic substances or beverages, including medications, or use alcohol while subject to being on-call in a paid status. An employee who has a confirmed alcohol concentration of 0.02 or greater, but less than 0.04, on an evidentiary breath testing device, will result in removal from his/her position for eight (8) hours or until the employee tests below a concentration level of less then 0.02, whichever is sooner. The employee will be placed in a non-pay status for the period of non-availability. A confirmed alcohol concentration of 0.04 or greater is considered a positive alcohol test and will result in disciplinary action for violation of this Policy.

G. SAFETY-SENSITIVE FUNCTIONS

In addition to the District's drug and alcohol testing program, employees who perform safety-sensitive functions, including contractors performing safety-sensitive functions on behalf of the District on or off District property, are required to participate in the federally mandated drug and alcohol testing program.

A safety-sensitive function as defined by the FTA, is any duty related to the safe operation of mass transit service including the:

1. Operation of revenue service vehicles, in or out of service,
2. Operation of non-revenue service vehicles that require drivers to hold a Commercial Driving License (CDL),
3. Controlling the dispatch or movement of revenue service vehicles,
4. Maintenance of revenue service vehicles or equipment used in revenue service, including parts repair, rebuilding and overhaul, and
5. Carrying of a firearm for security purposes.

A safety sensitive employee is considered to be performing a safety sensitive function when he or she is actually performing, ready to perform, or immediately available to perform such functions.

Tri-Met has reviewed the actual duties performed by employees to determine which functions and positions are safety-sensitive.

A list of safety-sensitive positions is attached (Exhibit A). The list will be up-dated as necessary.

H. PRESCRIPTION DRUG USE

The appropriate use of legally prescribed drugs and nonprescription medication is not prohibited. However, it is the policy of the District that each safety sensitive employee must report the use of medically authorized drugs that may impair job performance or mental function to her/his immediate supervisor prior to performing safety-sensitive duties. Employees must provide proper written medical authorization to work from a physician or dentist when using such authorized drugs. It is the employee's responsibility to inform the physician of the employee's job duties and determine from the physician, or other health care professional, whether or not the prescribed drug may impair their job performance, or mental or motor function. Legally prescribed drugs must be reported on the Notification of Prescription Drug form and must include the patient's name, the substance name, the quantity and frequency to be taken, the period of authorization, and name of authorizing health care professional.

Any failure to report the use of such drugs, or failure to provide proper evidence of medical authorization, may result in disciplinary action.

I. COMPLIANCE WITH TESTING

Any employee or applicant who refuses to comply with a request for testing, who provides false information in connection with a test, who modifies or alters test forms, or who attempts to falsify test results through tampering, contamination, adulteration, or substitution will be removed from duty immediately or barred from employment.

Refusal will include:

- an inability to provide a specimen or breath sample without a valid medical reason (confirmed by a physician);
- tampering, adulterating, or substituting specimen;
- delaying arrival at a designated collection site;
- leaving the collection site prior to test completion;
- failure to permit an observed or monitored collection when required;
- failure to take a second test when required;
- failure to undergo a medical evaluation when required;
- failure to cooperate with any part of the testing process;
- once test in underway, failing to remain at site and provide a specimen;
- failure to sign Step 2 of alcohol test form; and
- leaving the scene of an accident without just cause prior to submitting to a test.

Such refusals will be treated as insubordination and recorded as a positive test. The employee will be referred to the substance abuse professional, and will be subject to disciplinary action up to and including discharge.

J. GENERAL PROVISIONS FOR DRUG AND ALCOHOL TESTING

In order to promote and maintain a drug and alcohol-free workplace, the District will utilize a program of drug and alcohol screening. It is the District policy that this program applies to all employees except where noted.

All drug and alcohol testing will be in accordance with 49 CFR Part 40 (Procedures for Transportation Workplace Drug Testing Programs Sections), and Part 655 (Prevention of Alcohol Misuse and Prohibited Drug Use in Transit Operations). These regulations may be viewed on Tri-Net or obtained from Station Managers, Rail and Bus Maintenance Managers, and Managers of Rail Transportation, Field Operations and Facilities Maintenance, collection personnel and the Safety Department.

1. TYPES OF TESTING

a. Post-Offer/Pre-Employment (Safety Sensitive Positions Only)

Following a conditional offer of employment, applicants for all safety-sensitive positions will undergo urine drug testing as a condition of employment. As mandated by the FTA, applicants will be screened for the presence of marijuana, cocaine, opiates, phencyclidine (PCP), and amphetamines. In addition, under Tri-Met authority, applicants will be required to provide a second urine specimen for Non-DOT testing. The second specimen will be tested, using an extended testing panel for the presence of the aforementioned drugs as well as barbiturates, benzodiozepenes, methadone, and propoxyphene. Applicants will be notified of the testing requirement during the application process. Failure to appear, failure to remain at site prior to commencement of test and aborting the collection before the test commences is not considered a refusal of a pre-employment test.

A verified negative test result is required prior to performing any safety-sensitive functions and is a condition of employment. If the test is cancelled, the applicant must re-take the test and pass before being hired.

Failure to pass will result in the disqualification of the applicant. Applicants who fail to pass the drug screen will not be permitted to reapply for any position within the District for one year and must provide proof of having successfully completed a referral, evaluation and treatment plan.

Current District employees transferring into safety sensitive positions will not be allowed to perform safety sensitive duties until the employee takes a pre-employment drug test with a verified negative result. Additionally, current District employees returning to a safety sensitive position after a period of 90 days or more, must take a pre-employment drug test with a verified negative result before performing safety sensitive duties.

b. Reasonable Suspicion

It is the District's policy that all employees are subject to fitness-for-duty evaluation consisting of a drug and alcohol test when there is reason to suspect the employee is under the influence of alcohol or drugs on duty. A referral for testing will be made when a trained supervisor can articulate and substantiate physical, behavioral and performance indicators of probable drug use or alcohol misuse by observing the appearance, behavior, speech or body odors of the employee.

The FTA drug testing regulations require that all supervisors must undergo a minimum of 60 minutes of training on the signs and symptoms of drug use before they are qualified to make a reasonable suspicion determination. A similar provision in the FTA alcohol testing regulation requires supervisors to undergo an additional 60 minutes of training on the signs and symptoms of alcohol misuse.

The District provides and encourages refresher training for supervisory personnel.

The FTA requires that all employees in safety-sensitive positions will be tested for on or off duty drug use when there is reasonable suspicion of such impairment or use. Reasonable suspicion testing of safety-sensitive employees must be based on specific, contemporaneous, articulable observations concerning the appearance, behavior, speech, body odors, or direct observations of drug or alcohol use. In accordance with District policy, employees in non-safety-sensitive positions may be subject to the same criteria as employees in safety-sensitive positions, except that employees in non-safety-sensitive positions shall only be tested for reasonable suspicion of on duty drug or alcohol use or impairment.

Testing under Tri-Met authority will be conducted as Non-DOT testing and on Non-DOT chain of custody forms. The same high standards in testing procedures will be maintained.

Upon conclusion of the specimen collection, employees will be required to make arrangements for their own transportation home. If necessary, the District will make arrangements and pay for transportation. Under no circumstance will the employee be permitted to operate a motor vehicle for the trip home.

c. Post-Accident

All surviving safety-sensitive employees who have a direct or possible involvement in an accident while in the course and scope of their employment will be tested for the presence of drugs and alcohol under any of the following circumstances:

- A fatality has occurred;
- An individual suffers injury requiring immediate medical attention away from the scene;
- A bus, van, or automobile suffers disabling damage and must be towed from the scene; or
- A rail car or trolley car is removed from revenue service

Employees involved in accidents must refrain from alcohol use for eight (8) hours following the accident or until an alcohol test is administered. Employees must remain readily available. Employees who leave the scene of an accident without authorization or cannot be located for testing following the accident will be considered to have refused the test and will be subject to discipline, up to and including discharge.

Post-accident testing is stayed while the employee assists at the scene of the accident. In the event the employee is hospitalized or treated for injury, the drug and alcohol screen will be ordered at the treating facility.

In accordance with the FTA regulations, post accident tests administered by a law enforcement agency will be accepted in lieu of the FTA mandated tests, when the District is unable to perform the required tests due to law enforcement agency requirements.

Additionally, it is District policy to test employees for the presence of drugs and alcohol under the following circumstances:

- The employee receives a citation under State or local law, which impacts public safety, while in the course and scope of their employment; or
- The employee is involved in an event which violates District rules or procedures which poses a threat to the safety of employees or to the public, or property, including, but not limited to, run-away vehicles, or allowing a vehicle to strike a fixed object.

All testing under the District's authority will be conducted as a Non-DOT test on Non-DOT chain of custody forms.

Upon conclusion of the specimen collection, employees will be required to make arrangements for their own transportation home. If necessary, the District will make arrangements and pay for transportation. Under no circumstance will the employee be permitted to operate a motor vehicle home.

d. Random (Safety-Sensitive Positions Only)

Random testing of safety-sensitive employees will be conducted in a manner consistent with the requirements of 49 CFR Part 655 (Prevention of Alcohol Misuse and Prohibited Drug Use in Transit Operations) and 49 CFR Part 40 (Procedures for Transportation Workplace Drug and Alcohol Testing Programs).

The District will maintain a listing of the names of all employees in safety-sensitive positions. During the calendar year, drug and alcohol tests will be administered to these employees on a random-selection basis. The District shall ensure that random drug and alcohol tests conducted will be unannounced, immediate and that the dates for administering random tests are spread reasonably throughout the calendar month and year. Testing will be conducted on all days and hours during which safety-sensitive work is performed. All random test notifications will occur while the employee is on the clock. In the event the random test collection extends beyond the end of the shift, the employee will be paid overtime for the additional time, in accordance with the Collective Bargaining Agreement. There is no discretion on the part of management or operations in the selection and notification of individuals for testing.

A computer based random number generator, which is a scientifically valid method, is used for random selections. All safety-sensitive employees shall have an equal chance of being selected each time selections are made.

The FTA random testing rate requirement is to annually complete drug tests equivalent to 50% of the number of safety-sensitive employees and complete alcohol tests equivalent to 10% of the number of covered employees. It is the District's policy that the number of safety-sensitive employees selected

annually for drug and alcohol testing will be equal to a rate of at least 50% of the total number of safety-sensitive employees subject to testing.

The FTA may increase or decrease the minimum annual percentage rate for random drug and alcohol testing. Any changes to this rate will be noted in future amendments.

e. Return-To-Duty

All employees who test positive for drugs and/or alcohol, and who are allowed to return to work, must be evaluated for drug and alcohol use by a Substance Abuse Professional (SAP), must complete all disciplinary actions, and must test negative prior to being released for duty as outlined in 49 CFR Part 40.

It is the goal of this Policy to prevent substance abuse and rehabilitate rather than terminate the employment of workers. However, all persons covered by this Policy should be aware that violations of the Policy will result in discipline, up to and including termination, or in not being hired.

f. Follow-up

Employees permitted to return to duty following a positive test for drugs and/or alcohol will be subject to unannounced follow-up testing as determined by the SAP. The testing will be in accordance with 49 CFR Part 40, subpart O and will be in addition to the employee's selection for testing under the random testing program.

2. METHODOLOGY

Procedures for specimen collection, chain of custody of specimens, laboratory analysis procedures, and quality control requirements will be in accordance with the United States Department of Health and Human Services *Mandatory Guidelines for Federal Workplace Drug Testing Programs, Final Guidelines*, and the provisions set forth in 49 CFR Part 40, <u>Procedures for Transportation Workplace Drug and Alcohol Testing Programs</u> to assure a high degree of accuracy and reliability.

3. SUBSTANCE ABUSE PROFESSIONAL EVALUATIONS

An employee who tests positive for drugs or alcohol or refuses a test, will be removed immediately from his or her safety-sensitive functions and evaluated by a District-designated Substance Abuse Professional (SAP). The SAP will evaluate each employee to determine what assistance the employee needs in resolving problems associated with substance abuse. The evaluation will consist of a clinical assessment, treatment recommendations, and referrals, as appropriate. At a minimum, the employee must participate in a substance abuse education and prevention class. The SAP will inform the District, in writing, of the clinical-assessment-based treatment recommendations, which must be complied with. In addition, the SAP will specify the duration and frequency of follow-up drug and/or alcohol tests. The SAP's evaluations, assessment, treatment recommendations, referrals and follow-up testing recommendations will be in accordance with 49 CFR Part 40.

The District has secured the services of a Licensed Clinical Social Worker (LCSW) to perform the SAP duties. This individual has knowledge of and clinical experience in the diagnosis and treatment of drug and alcohol related disorders. Information regarding the current SAP is available from the Designated Employee Representative (DER).

4. CONFIDENTIALITY

Confidentiality will be maintained throughout the drug and alcohol testing process. To assure confidentiality, all test results will be sent only to the DER by means of a secure communication system.

The Safety Office will maintain results in a medical file separate from the official personnel file.

The employee has an unqualified right, upon written request, to obtain copies of any records pertaining to his or her drug or alcohol tests.
Test results will be released without written consent only:

- to those District personnel directly involved in the decision for the tested employee's dismissal or disciplinary action;
- to the decision-maker in a lawsuit, grievance, or other proceeding initiated by or on the behalf of the employee tested;
- when an accident investigation is performed by the National Transportation Safety Board; or,
- when records are requested by the DOT or any DOT agency with regulatory authority, including the state rail fixed guideway systems oversight agency.

The District will carry out this policy in a manner that respects the dignity and confidentiality of those involved.

Records will be made available to a subsequent employer upon receipt of a written request from the employee. As directed by the specific, written consent of the employee, information regarding the employee's record will be released to an identified person.

5. NOTIFICATION OF CRIMINAL OR DRIVING WHILE INTOXICATED CONVICTION

The Drug Free Workplace Act of 1988 requires all employees to notify the Drug and Alcohol Program Coordinator of any conviction under a criminal drug statute for violations occurring on District property within five (5) days of conviction. Additionally, the District policy requires the employee to notify the Drug and Alcohol Program Coordinator of all convictions under a criminal drug statute for violations occurring off District property and of all moving violation causing the loss of driver's license by State or local law enforcement involving drugs or alcohol. This notification must occur within five (5) days of conviction or violation. Failure to report such conviction, or violation, will result in disciplinary action up to and including discharge. The District is a Drug Free employer.

K. EMPLOYEE ASSISTANCE PROGRAM

The District recognizes its commitment and its responsibility to its employees by seeking to provide, through the Employee Assistance Program (EAP) and/or Substance Abuse Professional (SAP), an opportunity for employees to deal with drug and alcohol-related problems. Any employee who voluntarily requests assistance in dealing with a personal drug and/or alcohol problem may do so through the EAP and/or SAP in complete confidence and without jeopardizing his/her employment with the District solely because of the request for assistance. Telephone numbers for the EAP and SAP are available from the DER and/or the Human Resource Department. Other treatment programs for drug and alcohol problems are available through the health and welfare providers selected by individual employees. The discontinuation of any involvement with alcohol or drugs is an essential requisite for participation in any treatment program.

Although employees are encouraged to receive help for drug or alcohol problems, participation in an Employee Assistance Program and/or SAP will not excuse an employee's failure to comply with the requirements of this Policy.

L. EDUCATION AND TRAINING

DOT/FTA regulations require that all supervisors of safety-sensitive employees receive a minimum of 60 minutes of instruction on the alcohol program and an additional 60 minutes on the drug program. Supervisors who make reasonable suspicion determinations must have training on physical, behavioral, and performance indicators of probable drug and alcohol misuse.

Safety-sensitive employees will receive at least 60 minutes of drug awareness training. This training includes information on the effects and consequences of prohibited drug use on personal health, safety, the work environment, and indicators of prohibited use. Employees will also receive information on the effects of alcohol misuse on personal health, safety, the work environment, and available methods of intervention.

It is the policy of the District that training and education programs will be made available to all District employees and Union officials.

M. DISCIPLINE

Any employee whose conduct is found to be in violation of this Policy will be subject to disciplinary action, including immediate suspension or termination. Performance and other employment factors, and the nature of the violation will be taken into consideration in determining the degree of disciplinary action. Represented employees will be disciplined in accordance with the Collective Bargaining Agreement. All disciplinary action will be reviewable through the grievance procedures in the Collective Bargaining Agreement.

With respect to non-represented individuals, management shall have sole discretion to determine the appropriate disciplinary action for violation of this Policy.

N. RETURN-TO-WORK REQUIREMENTS

Prior to being allowed to return to work, all employees that test positive for drugs or alcohol, as defined under the terms of this Policy, and who, under the discipline policy, are allowed to return to work, will be required to successfully complete the following:

1. Meet with a Substance Abuse Professional (SAP) for assessment.
2. Abide by the treatment recommendations made by the Substance Abuse Professional (SAP), including successful completion of any treatment program or substance abuse prevention class, as applicable, and monitoring for a minimum of one year by the SAP to assure compliance with the aftercare plan.
3. Complete suspensions, as they may apply, consistent with the Collective Bargaining Agreement.
4. Undergo return-to-duty drug and alcohol tests. A verified negative result must be obtained before the employee will be permitted to return to work.
5. Complete a Return-To-Work Agreement, in conjunction with the employee's manager, outlining the terms for returning to work. The Agreement will be based in part on the SAP's terms of compliance. At a minimum the Return-to-Work Agreement will include the following requirements:
   a) Successful compliance with, and completion of the treatment program and/or substance abuse prevention class, as applicable; and
   b) Compliance with the after-care plan; and
   c) Participation in, and compliance with, the requirements of a follow-up testing program;

d) Immediate termination following a positive drug or alcohol test under any testing circumstances within the Return-to-Work Agreement time period. For the purposes of the Return-to-Work Agreement, a positive test is any confirmed alcohol concentration of .02 or greater; refusal to test or any confirmed positive drug test, verified by a Medical Review Officer (MRO); and

e) Employee signature on the Return-To-Work agreement acknowledging the acceptance and understanding of the conditions set forth within the agreement, in consideration of continued employment.

Failure to sign the Return-to-Work Agreement or failure to adhere to the any of the aforementioned requirements will result in termination of the employee.

O. MODIFICATIONS

The Designated Employer Representative (DER) is authorized and directed to promulgate modifications, amendments and revisions to the Tri-Met Drug and Alcohol Abuse Program and to enact any policies as may be necessary to ensure Tri-Met's compliance with laws and regulations affecting drug and alcohol matters.

P. PROGRAM ADMINISTRATION

The Safety Office is responsible for administering the Drug and Alcohol Abuse Policy and with certifying compliance with the FTA substance abuse program requirements. Any questions about the Policy, testing program or the drug and alcohol misuse prevention program may be addressed to the Manager, System Safety Programs at (503) 962-4943, or the Designated Employer Representative (DER) at (503) 962-4937.

The DER is knowledgeable about the DOT and FTA regulations, company policies and internal procedures. The DER is accessible to collection site personnel, Breath Alcohol Technicians (BAT), and Medical Review Officers (MRO) and is prepared to address drug and alcohol testing issues, make decisions, and provide direction in a timely manner. The DER has the authority to take necessary and immediate actions (directly or through the employee's direct supervisor) to remove employees from safety-sensitive duties, send employees for retests, and to direct the actions of service agents.

Q. BOARD APPROVAL

This policy has been approved and adopted by the Tri-Met Board of Directors.

RESOLUTION 02-03-20

RESOLUTION OF THE TRI-COUNTY METROPOLITAN TRANSPORTATION DISTRICT OF OREGON (TRI-MET) ADOPTING A A REVISED DRUG AND ALCOHOL ABUSE POLICY

WHEREAS, the Federal Transit Administration (FTA) requires all fund recipients to implement a drug and alcohol abuse policy in accordance with FTA regulations; and

WHEREAS, the FTA regulations require that a fund recipient's local governing board adopt the recipient's drug and alcohol abuse policy; and

WHEREAS, the Tri-Met Board of Directors (Board) approved and adopted Tri-Met's Drug and Alcohol Abuse Policy (Policy) on December 21, 1994; and subsequently revised the Policy on October 27, 1999; and

WHEREAS, Tri-Met desires to revise the October 27, 1999 Policy as set forth on the attached and incorporated Exhibit A;

NOW, THEREFORE, BE IT RESOLVED:

That the Board hereby approves and adopts the revised Tri-Met Drug and Alcohol Policy as set forth on the attached and incorporated Exhibit A.

Dated: March 27, 2002

_____
Presiding Officer

Attest:

_____
Recording Secretary

Approved as to Legal Sufficiency:

_____
Legal Department

Exhibit A. Tri-Met DOT/FTA-Defined Safety-Sensitive Positions and Codes

Tri-Met DOT/FTA-Defined Safety Sensitive Positions	Position Codes
Apprentice Vehicle Mechanic	0534
Apprentice Mechanic	0934
Assistant Supervisor	0529
Assistant Supervisor	0930
Assistant Supervisor	0964
Assistant Supervisor/Signals	0556
Assistant Supervisor/Track	0564
Assistant Supervisor/Traction PWR	0566
Bus Operator	0880
Dispatcher	0836
Helper	0533
Journeyman Mechanic	0931
Laborer/MOW	0561
Lead Road Supervisor	0839
LRT Lift/Fare Equipment Technician	0542
LRV Mechanic	0551
LRV Operator	0580
Maintenance Helper	0933
Maintenance Trainer	0918
Mini-Run Operator	0881
Plant Maintenance Mechanic	0557
Plant Maintenance Mechanic	0968
Power Maintainer	0531
Pressure Washer	0537
Rail/Controller/Supervisor	0536
Rail Signals Technician	0541
Rail Transportation Training Supervisor	0582
Road Supervisor	0834
Signal Maintainer Apprentice	0546
Spotter	0936
Tire Servicer	0941
Track Maintenance Technician	0540
Traction Overhead Technician	0547
Traction Power Substation	0545
Training Supervisor	0832

4. Des Moines Metropolitan Transit Authority (Iowa)

TABLE OF CONTENTS

Des Moines Metro Transit Authority
Substance Abuse Policy

1.0 Policy Statement

The Board of Trustees adopted the Des Moines Metro Transit Authority's Policy on Drug and Alcohol Abuse at its Board meeting on November 22, 1994, and revision of the original policy on November 18, 1997, August 22, 2000, and March 26, 2002. A copy of the latest Board approval is included in this policy. The Des Moines Metro Transit Authority (MTA) is dedicated to providing safe, dependable and economical transportation services to our transit system passengers. The MTA's employees are our most valuable resource, and it is our goal to provide a healthy, satisfying work environment, which promotes personal opportunities for growth. In meeting these goals, it is our policy to:

1. Assure that employees are not impaired in their ability to perform assigned duties in a safe, productive and healthy manner;
2. Create a workplace environment free from the adverse effects of drug abuse and alcohol misuse;
3. Prohibit the unlawful manufacture, distribution, dispensing, possession or use of controlled substances; and
4. To encourage employees to seek professional assistance any time personal problems, including alcohol or drug dependency, adversely affect their ability to perform their assigned duties.

2.0 Purpose

The purpose of this policy is to assure worker fitness for duty and to protect our employees, passengers and the public from the risks posed by the misuse of alcohol and use of prohibited drugs. This policy is also intended to comply with all applicable federal regulations governing workplace anti-drug and alcohol programs in the transit industry. The Federal Transit Administration (FTA) has published 49 CFR Part 655, as amended, that mandates urine drug testing and breath alcohol testing for safety-sensitive positions and prohibits performance of safety-sensitive functions when there is a positive test result. The U. S. Department of Transportation (DOT) has also published 49 CFR Part 40, as amended, that sets standards for the collection and testing of urine and breath specimens. In addition, the federal government published 49 CFR Part 29, "The Drug-Free Workplace Act of 1988," which requires the establishment of drug-free workplace policies and the reporting of certain drug-related offenses to the FTA. This policy incorporates those requirements for safety-sensitive employees and others when so noted.

3.0 Applicability

This policy applies to all safety-sensitive transit system employees, paid part-time employees, volunteers, contract employees and contractors when they are on transit property or when performing any transit-related, safety-sensitive business. This policy applies to off-site lunch periods or breaks when an employee is scheduled to return to work. Contract employees will not be permitted to conduct transit business if found to be in violation of this policy. Non-safety-sensitive employees are subject to this policy as noted.

In addition to being subject to all other elements of this policy, employees who perform "safety-sensitive functions" for MTA, as that term is defined in the FTA regulations (49 CFR Part 655), are subject to random drug and alcohol testing and other special requirements set forth in this policy. Generally, a safety-sensitive function occurs when an employee is performing, ready to perform or immediately available to perform any duty related to safe operation of mass transit services. The following are safety-sensitive functions:

1. Operation of a revenue service vehicle, whether or not such vehicle is in revenue service.
2. Controlling dispatch or movement of a revenue service vehicle.
3. Maintaining revenue service vehicles or equipment used in revenue service.
4. Operating a non-revenue service vehicle when required to be operated by a holder of a CDL.
5. Carrying a firearm for security purposes.
6. Supervising, where the supervisor performs any function listed in items 1-5 above.

MTA has reviewed the actual duties performed by employees in all job classifications to determine which employees perform safety-sensitive functions, and has determined which job functions may require the performance of safety-sensitive duties. An analysis will be performed if any new job classifications are developed to determine if the new job classifications should be considered safety-sensitive.

A list of safety-sensitive positions is included in this policy.

4.0 Prohibited Substances

Prohibited substances addressed by this policy include the following:

4.1 Illegally Used Controlled Substances or Drugs

Any illegal drug or any substance identified in Schedules I through V of Section 202 of the Controlled Substance Act (21 U.S.C. 812), and as further defined by 21 CFR 1300.11 through 1300.15. This includes, but is not limited to:

Marijuana Metabolite(1)	50 ng/ml	15 ng/ml
Cocaine Metabolite(2)	300 ng/ml	150 ng/ml
Amphetamines	1000 ng/ml	------------
Amphetamine	------------	500 ng/ml
Methamphetamine (3)	------------	500 ng/ml
Opiates	2000 ng/ml	------------
------------	------------	
Morphine	------------	2000 ng/ml
Codeine	------------	2000 ng/ml
Phencyclidine (PCP)	25 ng/ml	25 ng/ml

(1) Delta 9-tetrahydrocannabinol-9 carboxylic acid: (2) Benzoylecgonine; (3) Specimen must also include amphetamine at a concentration greater than or equal to 200 ng/ml.

Illegally used controlled substances include any drug not approved for medical use by the U.S. Drug Enforcement Administration or the U.S. Food and Drug Administration. Illegal use includes use of any illegal drug, misuse of legally prescribed drugs, and use of illegally obtained prescription drugs.

4.2 Legal Drugs

The appropriate use of legally prescribed drugs and non-prescription medications is not prohibited. However, the use of any substance which carries a warning label that indicates that mental functions, motor skills, or judgment may be adversely affected must be discussed by employees with their appropriate health care professional before performing work-related duties. Educational information regarding prescription and over-the-counter medications should be obtained from either a health care professional or pharmacist. Employees are urged strongly to seek and obtain medical advice prior to using prescription or over-the-counter drugs that may adversely affect his/her ability to safely operate or maintain vehicles.

A legally prescribed drug means that the individual has a prescription or other written approval from a physician for the use of a drug in the course of medical treatment. If the employee tests positive for drugs, he/she must provide within 24 hours a valid prescription. A valid prescription includes the patient's name, the name of the substance, quantity/amount to be taken, and the time period of the authorization. The misuse or abuse of legal drugs while performing transit business, in uniform or on transit property, is prohibited.

4.3 Alcohol

The use of beverages containing alcohol or substances including any medication, mouthwash, food, candy or any other substance such that alcohol is present in the body while performing transit business is prohibited. The concentration of alcohol is expressed in terms of grams of alcohol per 210 liter of breath as measured by a breath-testing device.

5.0 Prohibited Conduct

5.1 Manufacture, Trafficking, Possession and Use

All transit system employees are prohibited from engaging in the unlawful manufacture, distribution, dispensing, possession or use of prohibited substances on transit authority premises, in transit vehicles, in uniform, or while on transit authority business. Employees who violate this provision will be terminated. Law enforcement shall be notified, as appropriate, where criminal activity is suspected.

5.2 Intoxication/Under the Influence

Any safety-sensitive or non-safety-sensitive employee who is reasonably suspected of being intoxicated, impaired, under the influence of a prohibited substance, or not fit for duty shall be suspended from job duties pending an investigation and verification of condition. Employees who fail to pass a drug or alcohol test shall be removed from duty and referred to a Substance Abuse Professional (SAP). Failure of an employee to obtain a SAP evaluation and/or failure to follow the SAP's recommended treatment plan will be cause for termination of employment. A drug or alcohol test is considered positive if the individual is found to have a quantifiable presence of a prohibited substance in the body above the minimum thresholds defined in 49 CFR Part 40, as amended. Non-safety-sensitive employees are exempt under FTA regulations, but are governed under the MTA's own policy authority as noted.

5.3 Alcohol Use

No safety-sensitive or non-safety-sensitive employee should report for duty or remain on duty when his/her ability to perform assigned duties is adversely affected by alcohol or when his/her breath alcohol concentration is 0.04 or greater. No safety-sensitive or non-safety-sensitive employee shall use alcohol while on duty, in uniform, while performing safety-sensitive functions, or just before or just after (20 minutes) performing a safety-sensitive function. No safety-sensitive employee shall use alcohol within four hours of reporting for duty, or during the hours that they are on call. Violation of these provisions is prohibited and is cause for termination of employment. Non-safety-sensitive employees are exempt under FTA regulations, but are governed under the MTA's own policy authority as noted.

Not Negative Alcohol Test - (0.02 - 0.04) If an employee tests between 0.02 and 0.04 on an alcohol test, the employee will be removed from service for eight hours or unless a retest results in a concentration of less than 0.02. This absence will be considered an unexcused absence or loseout subject to MTA's disciplinary procedures.

5.4 Compliance with Testing Requirements

Under FTA guidelines, all safety-sensitive employees will be subject to urine drug testing and breath alcohol testing. Any safety-sensitive employee who refuses to comply with a request for testing shall be removed from duty, and consequences will be assessed. The MTA will consider the test refusal to be a positive test, and the employee will be provided with a list of Substance Abuse Professionals (SAP) for evaluation. Failure of an employee to obtain an SAP evaluation and/or failure to follow the SAP's recommended treatment plan will be cause for termination of employment. Any safety-sensitive employee who is suspected of providing false information in connection with a test, or who is suspected of falsifying test results through tampering, contamination, adulteration, or substitution will be required to undergo an observed collection. Verification of these actions will result in the employee's removal from duty and his/her employment terminated. Refusal can include an inability to provide a sufficient urine specimen or breath sample without a valid medical explanation, as well as, a verbal declaration, obstructive behavior, or physical absence resulting in the inability to conduct the test.

5.5 Treatment Requirements

All employees are encouraged to make use of the available resources for treatment of alcohol misuse, legal, and illegal drug use problems. Under certain circumstances, employees may be required to undergo treatment for substance abuse or alcohol misuse as explained in this policy. Any safety-sensitive employee who refuses or fails to comply with the SAP's requirements for treatment, after care or return-to-duty directives, will be cause for termination of employment. Non-safety-sensitive employees also must adhere to these same guidelines. Non-safety-sensitive employees are exempt under FTA guidelines, but adherence is regulated by the MTA's own policy authority. The employee's insurance provider will coordinate the cost of the treatment or rehabilitation services. Employees who do not have health insurance coverage are responsible for the entire cost of any recommended treatment or rehabilitation services.

5.6 Notifying MTA of Criminal Drug Conviction

Apart from FTA regulations, but under MTA's own authority, all employees are required to notify MTA of any criminal drug statute conviction for a violation within five working days after such conviction.

5.7 Proper Application of the Policy

The MTA is dedicated to assuring fair and equitable application of this substance abuse policy. Therefore, supervisors/managers are required to use and apply all aspects of this policy in an unbiased and impartial manner. Any supervisor/ manager who knowingly disregards the requirements of this policy, or who is found to deliberately misuse the policy in regard to subordinates, shall be subject to disciplinary action, up to and including termination of employment.

5.8 Voluntary Treatment

The Des Moines Metro Transit Authority encourages employees to seek treatment voluntarily. Any employee who comes forth and notifies the MTA of an alcohol or chemical abuse problem will be provided assistance. This assistance will include a mandatory referral to the MTA's Substance Abuse Professional (SAP) at the MTA's expense. Employees are encouraged but not mandated to follow the SAP's recommended treatment plan. An appropriate leave of absence may be granted for treatment and rehabilitation. Payment for treatment will be coordinated through the employee's health insurance provider. Employees who do not have health insurance coverage are responsible for the entire cost of any recommended treatment or rehabilitation services.

Voluntary requests for treatment must be made prior to any pending drug/alcohol test or disciplinary action. Employees will not be disciplined for requesting treatment, but will be expected to observe job performance standards and work rules as they apply to every employee. Any decision to seek help through the MTA will not interfere with an employee's eligibility for promotional opportunities. Confidentiality of information will be maintained at all times.

5.9 Non-Safety-Sensitive Employees

Apart from FTA regulations, but under MTA's own authority, non-safety-sensitive employees who have a positive drug or alcohol test will be referred to the MTA's Substance Abuse Professional (SAP) for assessment. The MTA will assist and encourage non-safety-sensitive employees to comply with the SAP's recommended treatment plan. Employees will be expected to observe job performance standards and work rules as they apply to every employee. Depending upon the non-safety-sensitive employee's job duties, the MTA reserves the right to remove the employee from his/her position and place the employee on an appropriate leave of absence. The MTA's Designated Employer Representative (DER) will determine if the non-safety-sensitive employee is capable of safely and satisfactorily performing his/her essential job functions as outlined in the employee's job description.

5.10   Confidentiality

The MTA affirms the need to protect individual dignity, privacy and confidentiality throughout the testing process. Laboratory reports or test results shall not appear in an employee's general personnel file. Information of this nature will be contained in a separate confidential medical folder that will be kept under the control of the Personnel Director. The reports or test results may only be disclosed without an employee's consent when:

1. The information is compelled by law or by judicial or administrative process;
2. The information has been placed at issue in a formal dispute between the employee and employer.

Employee must sign a separate release every time substance testing information is to be disclosed. The employee must sign releases anytime information is to be released to the employee, union representatives, subsequent employers, and to any other third party designated by the employee.

6.0 Testing Procedures

Urine drug testing and breath testing for alcohol may be conducted when circumstances warrant or as required by federal regulations. All safety-sensitive employees shall be subject to drug testing prior to employment, for reasonable suspicion, random, and following an accident as defined in Section 6.2, 6.3, 6.4, 6.5 and 6.6 of this policy. In addition, all safety-sensitive employees will be tested prior to returning to duty after failing a random drug or alcohol test. Follow-up testing will be conducted for a period of one to five years based on the SAP's recommendation, with at least six tests performed during the first year. Non-safety-sensitive employees will be subject to all testing except follow-up, return-to-duty and random testing under the MTA's own authority and not FTA regulations.

Testing shall be conducted in a manner to assure a high degree of accuracy and reliability and using techniques, equipment, and laboratory facilities that have been approved by the U. S. Department of Health and Human Services (DHHS). All testing will be conducted consistent with the procedures put forth in 49 CFR Part 40, as amended.

The drugs that will be tested for include marijuana, cocaine, opiates, amphetamines, and phencyclidine. An initial drug screen will be conducted on each urine specimen. For those specimens that are not negative, a confirmatory Gas Chromatography/Mass Spectometry (GC/MS) test will be performed. The test will be considered positive if the amounts present are above the minimum thresholds established in 49 CFR Part 40, as amended. In instances where there is reason to believe an employee is abusing a substance other than the five drugs listed above, apart from FTA regulations, MTA reserves the right to test for additional drugs under MTA's own authority using standard laboratory testing protocols.

All drug testing laboratory results will only be released to and reviewed by a qualified Medical Review Officer (MRO) in order to verify and validate test results. The MRO will release findings only to a Designated Employer Representative (DER). A MRO shall be a licensed physician who has knowledge of substance abuse disorders and has appropriate medical training to interpret and evaluate an individual's confirmed positive test result. Before verifying that an employee has a positive test result, the MRO is responsible for contacting any such employee, on a direct and confidential basis, to determine whether the employee wishes to discuss the test or present a legitimate explanation for the positive result. An MRO staff person may make the initial contact, but they are prohibited from gathering medical information. If, after reasonable efforts, the MRO is unable to reach the employee directly, the MRO may contact MTA's DER for assistance in contacting the employee. MTA's DER will take maximum precautions to preserve the confidentiality to the MRO contact.

If, after making all diligent and reasonable efforts, neither the MRO nor MTA's DER are able to contact the employee within ten (10) days of the date the MRO received the confirmed positive test result from the laboratory, the MRO may verify the test result as positive. The MRO may also verify the test result as positive if the employee does not contact the MRO within three (3) days of being contacted by MTA's DER or the employee expressly declines the opportunity to discuss the test result. The MRO may reopen the verification of positive test if the employee presents documentation of serious injury or illness or other circumstances that unavoidably prevented the employee from being contacted within the designated time period, and if the employee then presents a legitimate (in the MRO's opinion) explanation for the positive test, the MRO shall declare the test to be negative.

The MRO will review and interpret an individual's medical history, including any medical records and biomedical information provided; affording the individual an opportunity to discuss the test result; and decide whether there is a legitimate medical explanation for the result, including legally prescribed medication.

The MRO can declare a test invalid or canceled based on the regulations specified in 49 CFR Part 40. A canceled/invalid test is considered neither a positive nor a negative test. An example of a canceled test is a urine sample being rejected by the laboratory. The MRO shall cancel the test and report the cancellation and the reasons for it to the FTA, employer, and employee. A negative dilute specimen will not require a retest.

Tests for breath alcohol concentration will be conducted utilizing a National Highway Traffic Safety Administration (NHTSA) approved evidential breath-testing device (EBT) operated by a trained breath alcohol technician (BAT). All breath alcohol test results will be reported only by an MRO or BAT to a Designated Employer Representative (DER). If the initial test indicates an alcohol concentration of 0.02 or greater, a second test will be performed to confirm the results of the initial test. A safety-sensitive or non-safety-sensitive employee who has a confirmed alcohol concentration of greater than 0.02 but less than 0.04 will be removed from his/her position for eight hours unless a retest results in a concentration measure of less then 0.02. The inability to perform a safety-sensitive or non-safety-sensitive duty due to an alcohol test result greater than 0.02 but less than 0.04 will be considered an unexcused absence or loseout subject to MTA's disciplinary procedures. An alcohol concentration of 0.04 or greater will be considered a positive alcohol test and in violation of this policy and a violation of the requirements set forth in 49 CFR Part 655 for safety-sensitive employees. Any safety-sensitive or non-safety-sensitive employee that has a confirmed positive drug or alcohol test will be removed from his/her position, informed of educational and rehabilitation programs available, and referred to a Substance Abuse Professional (SAP) for assessment. Non-safety-sensitive employees are exempt under FTA regulations, but are governed under the MTA's own policy authority.

6.1 Compensation for Testing

The MTA will pay employees for drug or alcohol testing according to the following:

Paid Testing: (random, reasonable suspicion, follow-up, post injury and post-accident testing) Employees will be paid from the time they are notified of the testing and relieved of job duties or from the time they leave MTA property until such time as they are released by the supervisor escorting the employee.

In the case of alcohol testing at the MTA, the employee will be paid from the time they report to the appropriate office until they have completed the test.

Unpaid Testing: (pre-employment, pre-promotion or transfer, and return-to-work) Pre-employment, pre-promotion or transfer and return-to-work testing will not be compensable.

6.2 Split Specimen Testing

Any safety-sensitive or non-safety-sensitive employee who questions the results of a required drug test under paragraphs 6.2 through 6.8 of this policy may request that an additional test be conducted. This test must be conducted at a different DHHS-certified laboratory. The test must be conducted on the split sample that was provided by the employee at the same time as the original sample. All costs for such testing are paid by the employee unless the result of the split sample testing invalidates the result of the original test. Under MTA's authority, not the FTA's, the expense for the split specimen testing shall be borne by the employee and will be collected via a one-time payroll deduction upon receipt of bill of the split sample results. The method of collecting, storing, and testing the split sample will be consistent with the procedures set forth in 49 CFR Part 40, as amended. The employee's request for a split sample test must be made to the Medical Review Officer within 72 hours of notice of the original sample verified test result. Requests after 72 hours will only be accepted if the delay was due to documentable facts that were beyond the control of the employee. Non-safety-sensitive employees are exempt under FTA regulations, but adherence is regulated by the MTA's own policy authority.

6.3 Pre-Employment Testing

All safety-sensitive and non-safety-sensitive position applicants shall undergo urine drug testing immediately following the offer of employment or transfer into a safety-sensitive position. Receipt by the transit system of a negative drug test result is required prior to employment. Pre-employment drug tests may be administered only after the applicant has signed a consent form. Non-safety-sensitive applicants are tested apart from FTA regulations, but under MTA's own policy. Failure of a pre-employment drug test will disqualify an applicant for employment at the MTA for at least six months. The MTA will reconsider a safety-sensitive applicant's application for employment under the following conditions:

1. At least six months has lapsed between applications;
2. The applicant can show proof of successfully completing a substance abuse treatment program;
3. The applicant must pass a new drug test;
4. The applicant must be willing to be subjected to the random testing program devised for employees who have tested positive.

Should a safety-sensitive employee be unavailable to perform job duties for a period of ninety (90) days or more, the employee will be required to submit to a pre-employment drug screen prior to returning to their safety-sensitive job duties. Employee's transferring into a safety-sensitive position will be required to submit and pass a pre-employment drug test prior to the transfer.

6.4 Other Testing

Under MTA's own policy authority and not FTA's regulation all safety-sensitive and non-safety-sensitive employees may be required to submit to drug testing in conjunction with any required physical examination. Required physical examinations may include but are not limited to worker compensation injuries or any leave of absence of 30 days or more.

6.5 Reasonable Suspicion Testing

All safety-sensitive and non-safety sensitive employees may be subject to a fitness-for-duty evaluation, and urine and/or breath testing when there are reasons to believe that drug or alcohol use is adversely affecting job performance. Apart from FTA regulations, non-safety-sensitive employees are governed under MTA's own policy authority. A reasonable suspicion referral for testing will be made on the basis of specific, contemporaneous, and articulable observations concerning appearance, behavior, speech, or body odors of the employee consistent with possible drug use or alcohol misuse. An employee is reasonably suspected of prohibited drug use or alcohol misuse when a trained supervisor or other MTA authorized official can:

- Substantiate specific behaviors that may indicate drug use or alcohol misuse.
- Identify job performance problems that may indicate prohibited drug use or alcohol misuse.
- Actually observe physical indications that prohibited drug use or alcohol misuse may be occurring.

A supervisor or other MTA authorized official must make reasonable suspicion referrals. To make reasonable suspicion determinations, supervisors must be trained on the facts, circumstances, physical evidence, physical signs and symptoms, or patterns of performance and/or behaviors associated with drug use and/or alcohol misuse. One supervisor will complete the MTA's "Reasonable Suspicion" form, but two or more trained supervisors may participate in the reasonable suspicion determination process. A copy of the completed form will be provided to the employee Suspicion" form will be completed by one supervisor and a copy given to the employee.

6.6 Post-Accident Testing

All safety-sensitive employees will be required to undergo a urine drug test and breath alcohol test if they are involved in an FTA accident with a MTA transit vehicle (regardless of whether or not the vehicle is in revenue service). An FTA accident is defined as an occurrence associated with the operation of a revenue service vehicle that results in a fatality, in injuries requiring immediate transportation to a medical treatment facility; or one or more vehicles incur disabling damage that requires towing from the site. Safety-sensitive employees that are on duty in the vehicle and any safety-sensitive employee whose performance could have contributed to the accident will be tested. Accident does not necessarily mean collision. If an individual falls on a vehicle and needs to be transported to a hospital, then an accident has occurred and a post-accident test is required unless the driver can be completely discounted as a contributing factor to the accident. This definition only applies to non-fatal accidents. Fatal accidents will result in safety-sensitive employees being tested as outlined below.

Following an FTA accident, the safety-sensitive employee will be required to submit to a drug and alcohol test. Post-Accident testing is stayed while an employee assists in resolution of the accident or receives medical attention following the accident. However, employees must remain readily available during the time periods stated below. Post-accident testing will be done as soon as possible, and no later than (8) eight hours after the accident for alcohol testing and (32) thirty-two hours after the accident for drug testing. An employee involved in an accident must not use alcohol until after the employee undergoes alcohol testing or eight hours have elapsed, which ever comes first.

Nothing in this policy shall be construed to require the delay of necessary medical attention for the injured following an accident or to prohibit an employee from leaving the scene of an accident for the period necessary to obtain assistance in responding to the accident or to obtain necessary emergency medical care. However, any employee who under the above circumstance fails to remain available for drug and alcohol testing (including notifying MTA of his/her location), or who otherwise leaves the scene of the accident without appropriate authorization prior to drug and alcohol testing, will be considered to have refused the test.

49 CFR Part 40 allows the MTA to acquire post-accident test results obtained by Federal, State, or local law enforcement personnel in instances where the MTA is unavailable to perform post-accident testing. The results of a blood, urine or breath test for the use of prohibited drugs and alcohol misuse, conducted by Federal, State or local officials having independent authority for the test shall be considered to meet the FTA requirements provided such tests conform to the applicable Federal, State or local testing requirements and that the test results are obtained by the MTA.

6.7 Random Testing

In accordance with 49 CFR Part 655, employees in safety-sensitive positions will be subjected to random, unannounced testing. The selection of safety-sensitive employees for random drug and alcohol testing will be made using a scientifically-valid method that ensures each covered employee that they will have an equal chance of being selected each time selections are made. The random tests will be unannounced and spread throughout the year. The FTA determines the testing percentages annually. All safety-sensitive employees will be placed in a common selection pool. Each employee in this pool will be matched with a unique random selection number. Through the use of a computer-based random number generation program, the required number of persons will be selected for each testing cycle throughout the year. All employees in the pool will remain in the random selection pool at all times throughout the year regardless of whether or not they have been previously selected. Employees who are not available for testing during the testing period will be removed from the random pool prior to the random selection drawing occurring. The MTA's Personnel Director or DER will access the selection pool numbers. Notification will be made to those who must submit a specimen or complete an alcohol breath test. The test may be completed prior to, during or after the employee's work shift. The employee will be immediately escorted to the medical facility for the test. As soon as the urine specimen is collected or breath test is completed the employee will be required to return to work, unless the breath test is not negative.

6.8 Return-To-Duty Testing

All safety-sensitive employees who previously tested positive on a random drug or alcohol test must test negative (below 0.02 for alcohol) and be evaluated and released to duty by the Substance Abuse Professional before returning to work. If an employee refuses the return-to-duty test, he/she will be considered as having a second positive drug or alcohol test and his/her employment with the MTA will be terminated.

6.9 Follow-Up Testing

Safety-sensitive employees that have tested positive on a random test will be required to undergo frequent, unannounced random urine and/or breath testing following their return to duty after a positive drug/alcohol test and treatment. The follow-up testing will be performed for a period of one to five years based on the SAP's recommendations, however, a minimum of six tests to be performed the first year.

7.0 Employment Assessment

Any safety-sensitive employee, who tests positive for the presence of illegal drugs or alcohol above the minimum thresholds set forth in 49 CFR Part 40, as amended, will be referred for evaluation to a Substance Abuse Professional (SAP). A SAP is a licensed or certified physician, psychologist, social worker, employee assistance professional or addiction counselor with knowledge of and clinical experience in the diagnosis and treatment of alcohol or drug-related disorders. The SAP will evaluate each employee to determine what assistance, if any, the employee needs in resolving problems associated with prohibited drug use or alcohol misuse. If a safety-sensitive employee is allowed to return to duty, he/she must properly follow the rehabilitation program prescribed by the SAP, he/she must have a negative return-to-duty drug or alcohol test, and can be subject to unannounced follow-up tests for a period of one to five years. At least six follow-up tests are required in the first year following treatment. The employee's insurance provider will coordinate the cost of treatment or rehabilitation services. Employees who do not have health coverage are responsible for the entire cost of any treatment or rehabilitation services.

7.1 Consequences of a Positive Test

Effective April 15, 2002, the MTA will institute and maintain a zero tolerance policy for the following types of tests: Pre-employment, post-accident, and reasonable suspicion. A verified positive test for either post-accident, or reasonable suspicion will result in an employee's immediate termination of employment with the MTA.

The MTA will allow employees the ability to continue employment or what is considered a second chance for **random** tests only. Following a verified positive random test, the employee will be required to adhere to sections 6.8 and 6.9 of this policy. An employee who tests positive on a follow-up test following a positive random will be immediately discharged. Employees who test positive under random testing and subsequently returns to safety-sensitive duty will not be allowed to bid on or drive designated contracted school routes.

8.0 Re-Entry Conditions

Safety-sensitive employees who re-enter the workforce after a confirmed positive test must agree to re-entry conditions. Those conditions may include (but are not limited to):

1. A release to work statement from the Substance Abuse Professional.
2. A negative test for drugs and/or alcohol.
3. An employee signed agreement to unannounced frequent follow-up testing for a period of one to five years with at least six tests performed the first year.
4. An employee signed agreement to follow specified after-care requirements with the understanding that violation of the re-entry conditions is grounds for termination of employment.

If an employee has a **second positive** drug/alcohol test during the five-year period following a previously confirmed positive test, their employment with the MTA will be immediately terminated.

9.0 Drug and Alcohol Program Manager (DAPM) and Designated Employer Representative (DER)

Any questions regarding this policy or any other aspect of MTA's substance abuse program should be addressed to the following transit system representatives:

Drug and Alcohol Program Manager and Designated Employer Representative:

Name:	Debbie Wainwright
Title:	Personnel Director
Address:	1100 MTA Lane, Des Moines, IA 50309
Telephone Number:	(515) 283-8111
FAX Number:	(515) 283-8135

Assistant Drug and Alcohol Program Manager and Designated Employer Representative:

Name:	Donna Grange
Title:	Director of Operations - Paratransit
Address:	1100 MTA Lane, Des Moines, IA 50309
Telephone Number:	(515) 283-8111
FAX Number:	(515) 283-8135

A complete copy of regulation 49 CFR Part 40, as amended, is available for review in the Personnel Department.

Medical Review Officers:

Name:	Dr. David Berg
Title:	Physician
Address:	2100 Dixon, Suite 3
	Des Moines, IA 50316
Telephone Number:	(515) 265-1020

Name:	Dr. Anthony J. Sciorrotta
Title:	Physician
Address:	717 Lyon St., Suite D
	Des Moines, IA 50309
Telephone Number:	(515) 288-2269

Employee Assistance Program:

Name:	Employee & Family Resources
Address:	Ins. Exchange Bldg., 505 Fifth Ave., Suite 600
	Des Moines, IA 50309
Telephone Number:	(515) 244-6090

Substance Abuse Professionals

SAPs:	Tom Reynolds or Mark Eikenberry
Name:	Employee & Family Resources
Address:	Ins. Exchange Bldg., 505 Fifth Ave, Suite 600
	Des Moines, IA 50309
Telephone Number:	(515) 244-6090

Direct any questions regarding substance abuse to the following crisis hotline:

Foundation Two Crisis Line   1-800-332-4224

Des Moines Metro Transit Authority
Safety-Sensitive Positions
Revised March 1, 2002

Transportation:

Fixed Route Bus Operator (Full-Time)
Fixed Route Bus Operator (Part Time)
Fixed Route Dispatcher
Fixed Route Supervisor

Paratransit:

Paratransit Bus Operator (Full-Time)
Paratransit Bus Operator (Part-Time)
Paratransit Dispatcher (Full-Time)
Paratransit Dispatcher (Part-Time)
Paratransit Route Supervisor
Paratransit Scheduler

Maintenance:

Mechanic
Maintenance Director
Tireperson
Utility Person
Service/Cleaner (Full-Time)
Service/Cleaner (Part-Time)

Board Resolution

The Board of Trustees of the Des Moines Metropolitan Transit Authority hereby adopts the following resolution:

Substance Abuse Policy Statement Resolution

The Board of Trustees adopted the Des Moines Metropolitan Transit Authority's Policy on Drug and Alcohol Abuse at its board meeting on November 22, 1994, and revision of the original policy on November 18, 1997, August 22, 2000. A copy of the latest board approval is included in this policy. The Des Moines Metropolitan Transit Authority (MTA) is dedicated to providing safe, dependable and economical transportation services to our transit system passengers. MTA employees are our most valuable resource, and it is our goal to provide a healthy, satisfying work environment, which promotes personal opportunities for growth. In meeting these goals, it is our policy to:

1. Assure that employees are not impaired in their ability to perform assigned duties in a safe, productive and healthy manner.

2. Create a workplace environment free from the adverse effects of drug abuse and alcohol misuse.

3. Prohibit the unlawful manufacture, distribution, dispensing, possession or use of controlled substances.

4. Encourage employees to seek professional assistance anytime personal problems, including alcohol or drug dependency, adversely affects their ability to perform their assigned duties.

Signed by Chair Jacqueline Easley, this _____ day of March, 2002.

_____
Jacqueline Easley
Chair
Des Moines Metropolitan Transit Authority

5. Ohio Department of Transportation

TABLE OF CONTENTS

DRUG AND ALCOHOL TESTING POLICY

Adopted _____, 2001

Underlined text = Transit Authority requirements
Regular text = FTA requirements

> Insert name of transit agency in the blanks.

A. PURPOSE

The_____provides public transit and paratransit services for the residents _____. Part of our mission is to ensure that this service is delivered safely, efficiently, and effectively by establishing a drug and alcohol-free work environment, and to ensure that the workplace remains free from the effects of drugs and alcohol in order to promote the health and safety of employees and the general public. In keeping with this mission, _____declares that the unlawful manufacture, distribution, dispense, possession, or use of controlled substances or misuse of alcohol is prohibited for all employees.

> If your company policy is zero tolerance, state so on this page.

Additionally, the purpose of this policy is to establish guidelines to maintain a drug and alcohol-free workplace in compliance with the Drug-Free Workplace Act of 1988, and the Omnibus Transportation Employee Testing Act of 1991. This policy is intended to comply with all applicable Federal regulations governing workplace anti-drug and alcohol programs in the transit industry. Specifically, the Federal Transit Administration (FTA) of the U.S. Department of Transportation has published 49 CFR Part 655, as amended, that mandates urine drug testing and breath alcohol testing for safety-sensitive positions, and prohibits performance of safety-sensitive functions when there is a positive test result. The U. S. Department of Transportation (USDOT) has also published 49 CFR Part 40, as amended, that sets standards for the collection and testing of urine and breath specimens.

> All **Underlined** sections are suggested employer provisions and not required by the FTA. Transit system's must decide if the sections are to be deleted, if they remain, or if the provisions need to be changed to reflect current transit system policy, (i.e., disciplinary actions).

Any provisions set forth in this policy that are included under the sole authority of _____ and <u>are not</u> provided under the authority of the above named Federal regulations are underlined.

B. APPLICABILITY

This Drug and Alcohol Testing Policy applies to all safety-sensitive employees (full- or part-time) when performing any transit-related business. _____ employees that do not perform safety-sensitive functions are also covered under this policy under the sole authority of _____. A safety-sensitive function is any duty related to the safe operation of mass transit service including the operation of a revenue service vehicle (whether or not the vehicle is in revenue service), maintenance of a revenue service vehicle or equipment used in revenue service, security personnel who carry firearms, dispatchers or person controlling the movement of revenue service vehicles and any other transit employee who is required to hold a Commercial Drivers License. Maintenance functions include the repair, overhaul, and rebuild of engines, vehicles and/or equipment used in revenue service. A list of safety-sensitive positions who perform one or more of the above mentioned duties is provided in Attachment A. Supervisors are only safety sensitive if they perform one of the above functions.

C. DEFINITIONS

Accident means an occurrence associated with the operation of a revenue service vehicle even when not in revenue service in revenue service or which requires a Commercial Drivers License to operate, if as a result--

(1) A person dies;

(2) An individual suffers a bodily injury and immediately receives medical treatment away from the scene of the accident; or,

(3) One or more vehicles incurs disabling damage as the result of the occurrence and is transported away from the scene by a tow truck or other vehicle. For purposes of this definition, *disabling damage* means damage which precludes departure of any vehicle from the scene of the occurrence in its usual manner in daylight after simple repairs. Disabling damage includes damage to vehicles that could have been operated but would have been further damaged if so operated, but does not include damage which can be remedied temporarily at the scene of the occurrence without special tools or parts, tire disablement without other damage even if no spare tire is available, or damage to headlights, taillights, turn signals, horn, mirrors or windshield wipers that makes them inoperative.

Adulterated specimen. A specimen that contains a substance that is not expected to be present in human urine, or contains a substance expected to be present but is at a concentration so high that it is not consistent with human urine.

Alcohol means the intoxicating agent in beverage alcohol, ethyl alcohol, or other low molecular weight alcohols contained in any beverage, mixture, mouthwash, candy, food, preparation or medication.

Alcohol Concentration is expressed in terms of grams of alcohol per 210 liters of breath as measured by an evidential breath testing device.

Canceled Test is a drug test that has been declared invalid by a Medical Review Officer. A canceled test is neither positive nor negative.

Covered Employee means an employee who performs a safety-sensitive function including an applicant or transferee who is being considered for hire into a safety-sensitive function (See Attachment A for a list of covered employees), and other employees, applicants, or transferee that will not perform a safety-sensitive function but falls under the policy of the company's own authority.

Designated Employer Representative (DER) An employee authorized by the employer to take immediate action to remove employees from safety-sensitive duties and to make required decisions in testing. The DER also receives test results and other communications for the employer, consistent with the requirements of 49 CFR Parts 40 and 655.

Department of Transportation (DOT) Department of the federal government which includes the US Coast Guard, Federal Transit Administration, Federal Railroad Administration, Federal Highway Administration, Federal Motor Carrier Safety Administration, Research and Special Programs, and the Office of the Secretary of Transportation.

Dilute specimen. A specimen with creatinine and specific gravity values that are lower than expected for human urine.

Disabling damage means damage which precludes departure of any vehicle from the scene of the occurrence in its usual manner in daylight after simple repairs. Disabling damage includes damage to vehicles that could have been operated but would have been further damaged if so operated, but does not include damage which can be remedied temporarily at the scene of the occurrence without special tools or parts, tire disablement without other damage even if no spare tire is available, or damage to headlights, taillights, turn signals, horn, mirrors or windshield wipers that makes them inoperative.

Evidentiary Breath Testing Device (EBT) A Device approved by the NHTSA for the evidential testing of breath at the 0.02 and the 0.04 alcohol concentrations. Approved devices are listed on the National Highway Traffic Safety Administration (NHTSA) conforming products list.

Medical Review Officer (MRO) means a licensed physician (medical doctor or doctor of osteopathy) responsible for receiving laboratory results generated by the drug testing program who has knowledge of substance abuse disorders, and has appropriate medical training to interpret and evaluate an individual's confirmed positive test result, together with his/her medical history, and any other relevant bio-medical information.

Negative Dilute A drug test result which is negative for the five drug/drug metabolites but has a specific gravity value lower than expected for human urine.

Negative test result for a drug test means a verified presence of the identified drug or its metabolite below the minimum levels specified in 49 CFR Part 40, as amended. An alcohol concentration of less than 0.02 BAC is a negative test result.

Non-negative test result is a test result found to be adulterated, substitute, invalid, or positive for drug/drug metabolites.

Performing (a safety-sensitive function) means a covered employee is considered to be performing a safety-sensitive function and includes any period in which he or she is actually performing, ready to perform, or immediately available to perform such functions.

Positive test result for a drug test means a verified presence of the identified drug or its metabolite at or above the minimum levels specified in 49 CFR Part 40, as amended. A positive alcohol test result means a confirmed alcohol concentration of 0.04 BAC or greater.

Prohibited drug means marijuana, cocaine, opiates, amphetamines, or phencyclidine at levels above the minimum thresholds specified in 49 CFR Part 40, as amended.

Revenue Service Vehicles include all transit vehicles that are used for passenger transportation service or that require a CDL to operate. Include all ancillary vehicles used in support of the transit system.

Safety-sensitive functions include (a) the operation of a transit revenue service vehicle even when the vehicle is not in revenue service; (b) the operation of a non-revenue service vehicle by an employee when the operation of such a vehicle requires the driver to hold a Commercial Drivers License (CDL); (c) maintaining a revenue service vehicle or equipment used in revenue service; (d) controlling the movement of a revenue service vehicle; and (e) carrying a firearm for security purposes.

Substance Abuse Professional (SAP) means a licensed physician (medical doctor or doctor of osteopathy) or licensed or certified psychologist, social worker, employee assistance professional, or addiction counselor (certified by the National Association of Alcoholism and Drug Abuse Counselors Certification Commission or by the International Certification Reciprocity Consortium/Alcohol and other Drug Abuse) with knowledge of and clinical experience in the diagnosis and treatment of drug and alcohol related disorders.

Substituted specimen. A specimen with creatinine and specific gravity values that are so diminished that they are not consistent with normal human urine.

Test Refusal   The following are considered a refusal to test if the employee:
- Fails to appear for any test (excluding pre-employment) within a reasonable time, as determined by the employer, after being directed to do so by the employer
- Fails to remain at the testing site until the testing process is complete;
- Fails to provide a urine or breath specimen for any drug or alcohol test required by Part 40 or DOT agency regulations;
- In the case of a directly observed or monitored collection in a drug test, fails to permit the observation or monitoring of your provision of a specimen
- Fails to provide a sufficient amount of urine or breath when directed, and it has been determined, through a required medical evaluation, that there was no adequate medical explanation for the failure
- Fails or declines to take a second test the employer or collector has directed you to take;
- Fails to undergo a medical examination or evaluation, as directed by the MRO as part of the verification process, or as directed by the DER as part of the ``shy bladder'' or "shy lung" procedures
- Fails to cooperate with any part of the testing process (e.g., refuse to empty pockets when so directed by the collector, behave in a confrontational way that disrupts the collection process).
- If the MRO reports that there is verified adulterated or substituted test result
- Failure or refusal to sign Step 2 of the alcohol testing form.

Verified negative test means a drug test result reviewed by a medical review officer and determined to have no evidence of prohibited drug use above the minimum cutoff levels established by the Department of Health and Human Services (HHS).

Verified positive test means a drug test result reviewed by a medical review officer and determined to have evidence of prohibited drug use above the minimum cutoff levels specified in 49 CFR Part 40 as revised.

Validity testing is the evaluation of the specimen to determine if it is consistent with normal human urine. The purpose of validity testing is to determine whether certain adulterants or foreign substances were added to the urine, if the urine was diluted, or if the specimen was substituted.

D. EDUCATION AND TRAINING

Every covered employee will receive a copy of this policy and will have ready access to the corresponding federal regulations including 49 CFR Parts 655 and 40, as amended. In addition, all covered employees will undergo a minimum of 60 minutes of training on the signs and symptoms of drug use including the effects and consequences of drug use on personal health, safety, and the work environment. The training also includes manifestations and behavioral cues that may indicate prohibited drug use.

All supervisory personnel or company officials who are in a position to determine employee fitness for duty will receive 60 minutes of reasonable suspicion training on the physical, behavioral, and performance indicators of probable drug use and 60 minutes of additional reasonable suspicion training on the physical, behavioral, speech, and performance indicators of probable alcohol misuse. Under the _____'s own authority, supervisory personnel will also be trained on how to intervene constructively, and how to effectively integrate an employee back into his/her work group following intervention and/or treatment. Information on the signs, symptoms, health effects, and consequences of alcohol misuse is presented in Attachment B of this policy.

E. PROHIBITED SUBSTANCES

Prohibited substances addressed by this policy include the following.

(1) Illegally Used Controlled Substance or Drugs Under the Drug-Free Workplace Act of 1988 any drug or any substance identified in Schedule I through V of Section 202 of the Controlled Substance Act (21 U.S.C. 812), and as further defined by 21 CFR 1300.11 through 1300.15 is prohibited at all times in the workplace unless a legal prescription has been written for the substance. This includes, but is not limited to: marijuana, amphetamines, opiates, phencyclidine (PCP), and cocaine, as well as any drug not approved for medical use by the U.S. Drug Enforcement Administration or the U.S. Food and Drug Administration. Illegal use includes use of any illegal drug, misuse of legally prescribed drugs, and use of illegally obtained prescription drugs. Also, the medical use of marijuana, or the use of hemp related products, as which cause drug or drug metabolites to be present in the body above the minimum thresholds is a violation of this policy.

Federal Transit Administration drug testing regulations (49 CFR Part 655) require that all covered employees be tested for marijuana, cocaine, amphetamines, opiates, and phencyclidine as described in Section H of this policy. Illegal use of these five drugs is prohibited at all times, and thus covered employees may be tested for these drugs anytime that they are on duty.

(2) Legal Drugs: The appropriate use of legally prescribed drugs and non-prescription medications is not prohibited. However, the use of any substance which carries a warning label that indicates that mental functioning, motor skills, or judgment may be adversely affected must be reported to a _____ supervisor and the employee is required to provide a written release from his/her doctor or pharmacist indicating that the employee can perform his/her safety-sensitive functions.

(3) Alcohol: The use of beverages containing alcohol (including any mouthwash, medication, food, candy) or any other substances such that alcohol is present in the body while performing safety-sensitive job functions is prohibited. An alcohol test can be performed on a covered employee under 49 CFR Part 655 just before, during, or just after the performance of safety-sensitive job functions. Under _____ authority, an alcohol test can be performed any time a covered employee is on duty.

F. PROHIBITED CONDUCT

(1) All covered employees are prohibited from reporting for duty or remaining on duty any time there is a quantifiable presence of a prohibited drug in the body above the minimum thresholds defined in 49 CFR PART 40, as amended.

(2) Each covered employee is prohibited from consuming alcohol while performing safety-sensitive job functions or while on-call to perform safety-sensitive job functions. If an on-call employee has consumed alcohol, they must acknowledge the use of alcohol at the time that they are called to report for duty. The covered employee will subsequently be relieved of his/her on-call responsibilities and subject to discipline.

(3) The Transit Department shall not permit any covered employee to perform or continue to perform safety-sensitive functions if it has actual knowledge that the employee is using alcohol.

(4) Each covered employee is prohibited from reporting to work or remaining on duty requiring the performance of safety-sensitive functions while having an alcohol concentration of 0.04 or greater regardless of when the alcohol was consumed.

(5) No covered employee shall consume alcohol for eight (8) hours following involvement in an accident or until he/she submits to the post-accident drug/alcohol test, whichever occurs first.

(6) No covered employee shall consume alcohol within four (4) hours prior to the performance of safety-sensitive job functions.

> The four hours may be increased under the company's own authority.

(7) _____, under its own authority also prohibits the consumption of alcohol all times employee is on duty, or anytime the employee is in uniform.

(8) Consistent with the Drug-Free Workplace Act of 1988, all _____ employees are prohibited from engaging in the unlawful manufacture, distribution, dispensing, possession, or use of prohibited substances in the work place including Transit Department premises, transit vehicles, while in uniform or while on _____ business.

G. DRUG STATUTE CONVICTION

Consistent with the Drug Free Workplace Act of 1998, all employees are required to notify the _____ management of any criminal drug statute conviction for a violation occurring in the workplace within five days after such conviction. Failure to comply with this provision shall result in disciplinary action as defined in Section Q.10 of this policy.

H. TESTING REQUIREMENTS

Analytical urine drug testing and breath testing for alcohol will be conducted as required by 49CFR part 40 as amended. All covered employees shall be subject to testing prior to employment, for reasonable suspicion, following an accident, and random as defined in Section K, L, M, and N of this policy. All covered employees who have tested positive for drugs or alcohol on a random, reasonable suspicion, or post-accident will be tested prior to returning to duty after completion of the Substance Abuse Professional's recommended treatment program and subsequent release to duty. Follow-up testing will also be conducted following return-to-duty for a period of one to five years, with at least six tests performed during the first year. The duration and frequency of the follow-up testing above the minimum requirements will be at the discretion of the Substance Abuse Professional.

> If you are a zero-tolerance company, restate it at the end of this section.

A drug test can be performed any time a covered employee is on duty. An alcohol test can be performed just before, during, or after the performance of a safety-sensitive job function. Under _____ authority, an alcohol test can be performed any time a covered employee is on duty.

All covered employees will be subject to urine drug testing and breath alcohol testing as a condition of ongoing employment with _____. Any safety-sensitive employee who refuses to comply with a request for testing shall be removed from duty and subject to discipline as defined in Section Q.3 of this policy. Any covered employee who is suspected of providing false information in connection with a drug test, or who is suspected of falsifying test results through tampering, contamination, adulteration, or substitution will be required to undergo an observed collection. Verification of the above listed actions will be considered a test refusal and will result in the employees removal from duty and disciplined as defined in Section Q.3 of this policy. Refer to Section C.3 for behavior that constitutes a refusal to test.

I. DRUG TESTING PROCEDURES

Testing shall be conducted in a manner to assure a high degree of accuracy and reliability and using techniques, equipment, and laboratory facilities which have been approved by the U.S. Department of Health and Human Service (HHS). All testing will be conducted consistent with the procedures set forth in 49 CFR Part 40, as amended. The procedures will be performed in a private, confidential manner and every effort will be made to protect the employee, the integrity of the drug testing procedure, and the validity of the test result.

The drugs that will be tested for include marijuana, cocaine, opiates, amphetamines, and phencyclidine. After the identity of the donor is checked using picture identification, a urine specimen will be collected using the split specimen collection method described in 49 CFR Part 40, as amended. Each specimen will be accompanied by a DOT Chain of Custody and Control Form and identified using a unique identification number that attributes the specimen to the correct individual. The specimen analysis will be conducted at a HHS certified laboratory. An initial drug screen and validity test will be conducted on the primary urine specimen. For those specimens that are not negative, a confirmatory Gas Chromatography/Mass Spectrometry (GC/MS) test will be performed. The test will be considered positive if the amounts of the drug(s) and/or its metabolites identified by the GC/MS test are above the minimum thresholds established in 49 CFR Part 40, as amended.

The test results from the HHS certified laboratory will be reported to a Medical Review Officer (MRO). An MRO is a licensed physician with detailed knowledge of substance abuse disorders and drug testing. The MRO will review the test results to ensure the scientific validity of the test and to determine whether there is a legitimate medical explanation for a confirmed positive, substitute, or adulterated test result. The MRO will attempt to contact the employee to notify the employee of the non-negative laboratory result, and provide the employee with an opportunity to explain the confirmed laboratory test result. The MRO will subsequently review the employee's medical history/medical records as appropriate to determine whether there is a legitimate medical explanation for a non-negative laboratory result. If no legitimate medical explanation is found, the test will be verified positive or refusal to test and reported to the _____ Drug and Alcohol Program Manager (DAPM). If a legitimate explanation is found, the MRO will report the test result as negative to the DAPM and no further action will be taken. If the test is invalid with out a medical explanation, a retest will be conducted under direct observation.

Any covered employee who questions the results of a required drug test under paragraphs L through P of this policy may request that the split sample be tested. The split sample test must be conducted at a second HHS-certified laboratory with no affiliation with the laboratory that analyzed the primary specimen. The test must be conducted on the split sample that was provided by the employee at the same time as the primary sample. The method of collecting, storing, and testing the split sample will be consistent with the procedures set forth in 49 CFR Part 40, as amended. The employee's request for a split sample test must be made to the Medical Review Officer within 72 hours of notice of the original sample verified test result. Requests after 72 hours will only be accepted at the discretion of the MRO if the delay was due to documentable facts that were beyond the control of the employee. _____ will ensure that the cost for the split specimen are covered in order for a timely analysis of the sample, however _____ will seek reimbursement for the split sample test from the employee.

If the analysis of the split specimen fails to confirm the presence of the drug(s) detected in the primary specimen, if the split specimen is not able to be analyzed, or if the results of the split specimen are not scientifically adequate, the MRO will declare the original test to be canceled and will direct _____ to retest the employee under direct observation.

The split specimen will be stored at the initial laboratory until the analysis of the primary specimen is completed. If the primary specimen is negative, the split will be discarded. If the primary is positive, the split will be retained for testing if so requested by the employee through the Medical Review Officer. If the primary specimen is positive, it will be retained in frozen storage for one year and the split specimen will also be retained for one year.

Observed collections:

Consistent with 49 CFR part 40, as amended, collection under direct observation (by a person of the same gender) with no advance notice will occur if:
    (1) The laboratory reports to the MRO that a specimen is invalid, and the MRO reports to _____ that there was not an adequate medical explanation for the result; or
    (2) The MRO reports to _____ that the original positive, adulterated, or substituted test result had to be cancelled because the test of the split specimen could not be performed.
    (3) The collector observes materials brought to the collection site or the employee's conduct clearly indicates an attempt to tamper with a specimen or
    (4) The temperature on the original specimen was out of range.

In addition, _____ may direct a collection under direct observation of an employee if the drug test is a return-to-duty test or a follow-up test.

J. ALCOHOL TESTING PROCEDURES

Tests for breath alcohol concentration will be conducted utilizing a National Highway Traffic Safety Administration (NHTSA)-approved Evidential Breath Testing device (EBT) operated by a trained Breath Alcohol Technician (BAT). Alcohol screening tests may be performed using a non-evidential testing device which is also approved by NHSTA. If the initial test indicates an alcohol concentration of 0.02 or greater, a second test will be performed to confirm the results of the initial test. The confirmatory test must occur on an EBT. The confirmatory test will be conducted at least fifteen minutes after the completion of the initial test. The confirmatory test will be performed using a NHTSA-approved EBT operated by a trained BAT. The EBT will identify each test by a unique sequential identification number. This number, time, and unit identifier will be provided on each EBT printout. The EBT printout, along with an approved alcohol testing form, will be used to document the test, the subsequent results, and to attribute the test to the correct employee. The test will be performed in a private, confidential manner as required by 49 CFR Part 40, as amended. The procedure will be followed as prescribed to protect the employee and to maintain the integrity of the alcohol testing procedures and validity of the test result.

An employee who has a confirmed alcohol concentration of 0.04 or greater will be considered a positive alcohol test and in violation of this policy. The consequences of a positive alcohol test are described in Section Q.4-5 of this policy. Even though an employee who has a confirmed alcohol concentration of 0.02 to 0.039 is not considered positive, the employee shall still be removed from duty for at least eight hours _or for the duration of the work day whichever is longer_ and will be subject to the consequences described in Section Q.9 of this policy. An alcohol concentration of less than 0.02 will be considered a negative test.

The Transit Department affirms the need to protect individual dignity, privacy, and confidentiality throughout the testing process. If at any time the integrity of the testing procedures or the validity of the test results is compromised, the test will be canceled. Minor inconsistencies or procedural flaws that do not impact the test result will not result in a cancelled test.

The alcohol testing form (ATF) required by 49 CFR Part 40 as amended, shall be used for all FTA required testing. Failure of an employee to sign step 2 of the ATF will be considered a refusal to submit to testing.

K. PRE-EMPLOYMENT TESTING

All applicants for covered transit positions shall undergo urine drug testing _and breath alcohol testing_ prior to performance of a safety-sensitive function.

 (1) All offers of employment for covered positions shall be extended conditional upon the applicant passing a drug _and alcohol test_ test. An applicant shall not be hired into a covered position unless the applicant takes a drug test with verified negative results, _and an alcohol concentration below 0.02._

 (2) A non-covered employee shall not be placed, transferred or promoted into a covered position until the employee takes a drug test with verified negative results _and an alcohol concentration below 0.02._

 (3) If an applicant fails a pre-employment drug or alcohol test, the conditional offer of employment shall be rescinded. Failure of a pre-employment drug and/or alcohol test will disqualify an applicant for employment for a period of at least one year. Evidence of the absence of drug dependency from a Substance Abuse Professional that meets with 49 CFR part 40 as amended and a negative pre-employment drug test _and an alcohol concentration below 0.02_ will be required prior to further consideration for employment. The cost for the assessment and any subsequent treatment will be the sole responsibility of the applicant.

 (4) When an employee being placed, transferred, or promoted from a non-covered position to a covered position submits a drug test with a verified positive result, _and an alcohol concentration below 0.02_ the employee shall be subject to disciplinary action in accordance with Section Q.4-5 and 9 herein.

 (5) If a pre-employment/pre-transfer test is canceled, _____ will require the applicant to take and pass another pre-employment drug test.

(6)   In instances where a covered employee is on extended leave for a period of 90 days or more regardless of reason, the employee will be required to take a drug *and alcohol* test under 49 CFR Part 655 and have negative test results prior to the conduct of safety-sensitive job functions.

(7)   An applicant with a dilute negative test result will be required to retest.

(8)   Applicants are required to report previous DOT covered employer drug and alcohol test results—Failure to do so will result in the employment offer being rescinded.

L.   REASONABLE SUSPICION TESTING

All _____ covered employees will be subject to a reasonable suspicion drug and/or alcohol test when there are reasons to believe that drug or alcohol use is impacting job performance and safety. Reasonable suspicion shall mean that there is objective evidence, based upon specific, contemporaneous, articulable observations of the employee's appearance, behavior, speech or body odor that are consistent with possible drug use and/or alcohol misuse. Reasonable suspicion referrals must be made by one supervisor who is trained to detect the signs and symptoms of drug and alcohol use, and who reasonably concludes that an employee may be adversely affected or impaired in his/her work performance due to possible prohibited substance abuse or alcohol misuse. A reasonable suspicion alcohol test can only be conducted just before, during, or just after the performance of a safety-sensitive job function. However, under _____ 's authority, a reasonable suspicion alcohol test may be performed any time the covered employee is on duty. A reasonable suspicion drug test can be performed any time the covered employee is on duty.

_____ shall be responsible for transporting the employee to the testing site. Supervisors should avoid placing themselves and/or others into a situation which might endanger the physical safety of those present. The employee shall be placed on administrative leave pending disciplinary action described in Section Q.4-5 and 9 of this policy. An employee who refuses an instruction to submit to a drug/alcohol test shall not be permitted to finish his or her shift and shall immediately be placed on administrative leave pending disciplinary action as specified in Section Q.3 of this policy.

A written record of the observations which led to a drug/alcohol test based on reasonable suspicion shall be prepared and signed by the supervisor making the observation prior to the release of the test results. This written record shall be submitted to the _____ management and shall be attached to the forms reporting the test results.

When there are no specific, contemporaneous, articulable objective facts that indicate current drug or alcohol use, but the employee (who is not already a participant in a treatment program) admits the abuse of alcohol or other substances to a supervisor in his/her chain of command, the employee shall be referred to the SAP for an assessment. _____ shall place the employee on administrative leave in accordance with the provisions set forth under Section Q.9 of this policy. Testing in this circumstance would be performed under the direct authority of the _____ . Since the employee self-referred to management, testing under this circumstance would not be considered a violation of this policy or a positive test result under Federal authority. However, self-referral does not exempt the covered employee from testing under Federal authority as specified in Sections L through N of this policy or the associated consequences as specified in Section Q.9.

M. POST-ACCIDENT TESTING

All covered employees will be required to undergo urine and breath testing if they are involved in an accident with a transit revenue service vehicle regardless of whether or not the vehicle is in revenue service that results in a fatality. This includes all surviving covered employees that are operating the vehicle at the time of the accident and any other whose performance cannot be completely discounted as a contributing factor to the accident.

In addition, a post-accident test will be conducted if an accident results in injuries requiring immediate transportation to a medical treatment facility; or one or more vehicles incurs disabling damage, unless the operators performance can be completely discounted as a contributing factor to the accident.

(1)   As soon as practicable following an accident, as defined in this policy, the transit supervisor investigating the accident will notify the transit employee operating the transit vehicle and all other covered employees whose performance could have contributed to the accident of the need for the test. The supervisor will make the determination using the best information available at the time of the decision.

(2)   The appropriate transit supervisor shall ensure that an employee, required to be tested under this section, is tested as soon as practicable, but no longer than eight (8) hours of the accident for alcohol, and within 32 hours for drugs. If an alcohol test is not performed within two hours of the accident, the Supervisor will document the reason(s) for the delay. If the alcohol test is not conducted within (8) eight hours, or the drug test within 32 hours, attempts to conduct the test must cease and the reasons for the failure to test documented.

(3)   Any covered employee involved in an accident must refrain from alcohol use for eight (8) hours following the accident, or until he/she undergoes a post-accident alcohol test.

(4)   An employee who is subject to post-accident testing who fails to remain readily available for such testing, including notifying a supervisor of his or her location if he or she leaves the scene of the accident prior to submission to such test, may be deemed to have refused to submit to testing.

(5)   Nothing in this section shall be construed to require the delay of necessary medical attention for the injured following an accident, or to prohibit an employee from leaving the scene of an accident for the period necessary to obtain assistance in responding to the accident, or to obtain necessary emergency medical care.

(6)   In the rare event that _____ is unable to perform an FTA drug and alcohol test (i.e., employee is unconscious, employee is detained by law enforcement agency), _____ may use drug and alcohol post-accident test results administered by local law enforcement officials in lieu of the FTA test. The local law enforcement officials must have independent authority for the test and the employer must obtain the results in conformance with local law.

N. RANDOM TESTING

All covered employees will be subjected to random, unannounced testing. The selection of employees shall be made by a scientifically valid method of randomly generating an employee identifier from the appropriate pool of safety-sensitive employees.

(1)   The dates for administering unannounced testing of randomly selected employees shall be spread reasonably throughout the calendar year.

(2)   The number of employees randomly selected for drug/alcohol testing during the calendar year shall be not less than the percentage rates established by Federal regulations for those safety-sensitive employees subject to random testing by Federal regulations. The current random testing rate for drugs established by FTA equals fifty percent of the number of covered employees in the pool and the random testing rate for alcohol established by FTA equals ten percent of the number of covered employees in the pool.

(3)   Each covered employee shall be in a pool from which the random selection is made. Each covered employee in the pool shall have an equal chance of selection each time the selections are made. Employees will remain in the pool and subject to selection, whether or not the employee has been previously tested. There is no discretion on the part of management in the selection and notification of the individuals who are to be tested.

(4)   Covered transit employees that fall under the Federal Transit Administration regulations will be included in one random pool maintained separately from the testing pool of employees that are included solely under _____ authority.

> **Random test pools can include any DOT covered employee. If you have both FTA and FMCSA covered employees, they can be in the same pool.**

(5)   Random tests can be conducted at any time during an employee's shift for drug testing. Alcohol random tests can be performed just before, during, or just after the performance of a safety sensitive duty. However, under the _____'s authority, a random alcohol test may be performed any time the covered employee is on duty. Testing can occur during the beginning, middle, or end of an employee's shift.

(6)   Employees are required to proceed immediately to the collection site upon notification of their random selection.

> **Each employer defines a reasonable time for reporting for a random test.**

O. RETURN-TO-DUTY TESTING

All covered employees who previously tested positive on a drug or alcohol test or refused a test, must test negative for drugs, alcohol (below 0.02 for alcohol), or both and be evaluated and released by the Substance Abuse Professional before returning to work. For an initial positive drug test a Return-to-Duty drug test is required and an alcohol test is allowed. For an initial positive alcohol test a Return-to-Duty alcohol test is required and a drug test is allowed. Following the initial assessment, the SAP will recommend a course of rehabilitation unique to the individual. The SAP will recommend the return-to-duty test only when the employee has successfully completed the treatment requirement and is known to be drug- and alcohol-free and there is no undo concerns for public safety.

> **If you are a zero-tolerance company, restate so before this section.**

P. FOLLOW-UP TESTING

Covered employees will be required to undergo frequent, unannounced drug and alcohol testing following their return-to-duty. The follow-up testing will be performed for a period of one to five years with a minimum of six tests to be performed the first year. The frequency and duration of the follow-up tests (beyond the minimums) will be determined by the SAP reflecting the SAP's assessment of the employee's unique situation and recovery progress. Follow-up testing should be frequent enough to deter and/or detect a relapse. Follow-up testing is separate and in addition to the random, post-accident, reasonable suspicion and return-to-duty testing.

Q. RESULT OF DRUG/ALCOHOL TEST

Any covered employee that has a verified positive drug or alcohol test will be removed from his/her safety-sensitive position, informed of educational and rehabilitation programs available, and referred to a Substance Abuse Professional (SAP) for assessment. No employee will be allowed to return to duty requiring the performance of safety-sensitive job functions without the approval of the SAP.

A positive drug and/or alcohol test will also result in disciplinary action as specified herein.

(1)   As soon as practicable after receiving notice of a verified positive drug test result, a confirmed alcohol test result, or a test refusal, the _____ Drug and Alcohol Program Manager will contact the employee's supervisor to have the employee cease performing any safety-sensitive function.

(2)   The employee shall be referred to a Substance Abuse Professional for an assessment. The SAP will evaluate each employee to determine what assistance, if any, the employee needs in resolving problems associated with prohibited drug use or alcohol misuse.

(3)   Refusal to submit to a drug/alcohol test shall be considered a positive test result and a direct act of insubordination and shall result in termination. A test refusal includes the following circumstances.

(a) A covered employee who consumes alcohol within eight (8) hours following involvement in an accident without first having submitted to post-accident drug/alcohol tests.

(b) A covered employee who leaves the scene of an accident without a legitimate explanation prior to submission to drug/alcohol tests.

(c) A covered employee who is suspected of providing false information in connection with a drug test.

(d) A covered employee who provides an insufficient volume of urine specimen or breath sample without a valid medical explanation. The medical evaluation shall take place within 5 days of the initial test attempt.

(e) A verbal or written declaration, obstructive behavior, or physical absence resulting in the inability to conduct the test within the specified time frame.

(f) A covered employee whose urine sample has been verified by the MRO as substitute or adulterated.

(g) A covered employee fails to appear for any test within a reasonable time, as determined by the employer, after being directed to do so by the employer

(h) A covered employee fails to remain at the testing site until the testing process is complete;

(i) A covered employee fails to provide a urine specimen for any drug test required by Part 40 or DOT agency regulations;

(j) A covered employee fails to permit the observation or monitoring of a specimen collection

(k) A covered employee fails or declines to take a second test the employer or collector has directed you to take;

(l) A covered employee fails to undergo a medical examination or evaluation, as directed by the MRO as part of the verification process, or as directed by the DER as part of the "shy bladder" or "shy lung" procedures

(m) A covered employee fails to cooperate with any part of the testing process (e.g., refuse to empty pockets when so directed by the collector, behave in a confrontational way that disrupts the collection process).

(n) Failure to sign Step 2 of the Alcohol Testing form

(4) For the first instance of a verified positive test from a sample submitted as the result of a random, drug/alcohol test ($\geq$ 0.04 BAC), disciplinary action against the employee shall include:

> *If your policy is zero tolerance this section must be removed.*

(a) Mandatory referral to Substance Abuse Professional for assessment, formulation of a treatment plan, and execution of a return to work agreement;

(b) Failure to execute, or remain compliant with the return-to-work agreement shall result in termination from   employment.

- ♦ Compliance with the return-to-work agreement means that the employee has submitted to a drug/alcohol test immediately prior to returning to work; the result of that test is negative; in the judgement of the SAP the employee is cooperating with his/her SAP recommended treatment program; and, the employee has agreed to periodic unannounced follow-up testing as defined in Section P of this policy;

(c) Refusal to submit to a periodic unannounced follow-up drug/alcohol test shall be considered a direct act of insubordination and shall result in termination.

(d) A periodic unannounced follow-up drug/alcohol test which results in a verified positive shall result in termination from   employment.

(5) The second instance of a verified positive drug or alcohol ($\geq$ 0.04 BAC) test result including a sample submitted under the random, reasonable suspicion, return-to-duty, or follow-up drug/alcohol test provisions herein shall result in termination from   employment.

(6) A verified positive post-accident, or reasonable suspicion drug and/or alcohol ($\geq$ 0.04) test shall result in termination.

(7) An alcohol test result of $\geq$0.02 to $\leq$ 0.039 BAC shall result in the removal of the employee from duty for eight hours or the remainder or the work day whichever is longer. The employee will not be allowed to return to safety-sensitive duty for his/her next shift until he/she submits to an alcohol test with a result of less than 0.02 BAC. If the employee has an alcohol test result of $\geq$ 0.02 to $\leq$ 0.039 two or more times within a six month period, the employee will be removed from duty and referred to the SAP for assessment and treatment consistent with Section Q.9 of this policy.

(8) The cost of any treatment or rehabilitation services will be paid directly by the employee or their insurance provider. The employee will be permitted to take accrued sick leave or administrative leave to participate in the SAP prescribed treatment program. If the employee has insufficient accrued leave, the

employee shall be placed on leave without pay until the SAP has determined that the employee has successfully completed the required treatment program and releases him/her to return-to-duty. Any leave taken, either paid or unpaid, shall be considered leave taken under the Family and Medical Leave Act.

    (9)   In the instance of a self-referral or a management referral, disciplinary action against the employee shall include:

        (a)   Mandatory referral to a Substance Abuse Professional for assessment, formulation of a treatment plan, and execution of a return to work agreement;

        (b)   Failure to execute, or remain compliant with the return-to-work agreement shall result in termination from   employment.

            ◆   Compliance with the return-to-work agreement means that the employee has submitted to a drug/alcohol test immediately prior to returning to work; the result of that test is negative; in the judgment of the SAP the employee is cooperating with his/her SAP recommended treatment program; and, the employee has agreed to periodic unannounced follow-up testing as defined in Section P of this policy;

        (c)   Refusal to submit to a periodic unannounced follow-up drug/alcohol test shall be considered a direct act of insubordination and shall result in termination.

        (d)   A self-referral or management referral to the SAP that was not precipitated by a positive test result does not constitute a violation of the Federal regulations and will not be considered as a positive test result in relation to the progressive discipline defined in Section Q.4-5 of this policy.

        (e)   Periodic unannounced follow-up drug/alcohol test conducted as a result of a self-referral or management referral which results in a verified positive shall be considered a positive test result in relation to the progressive discipline defined in Section Q.4-5 of this policy.

        (f)   A Voluntary Referral does not shield an employee from disciplinary action or guarantee employment with   .

        (g)   A Voluntary Referral does not shield an employee from the requirement to comply with drug and alcohol testing.

    (10)   Failure of an employee to report within five days a criminal drug statute conviction for a violation occurring in the workplace shall result in termination.

R. GRIEVANCE AND APPEAL

The consequences specified by 49 CFR Part 655 for a positive test or test refusal are not subject to arbitration.

S. PROPER APPLICATION OF THE POLICY

_____ is dedicated to assuring fair and equitable application of this substance abuse policy. Therefore, supervisors/managers are required to use and apply all aspects of this policy in an unbiased and impartial manner. Any supervisor/manager who knowingly disregards the requirements of this policy, or who is found to deliberately misuse the policy in regard to subordinates, shall be subject to disciplinary action, up to and including termination.

T. INFORMATION DISCLOSURE

Drug/alcohol testing records shall be maintained by the _____ Drug and Alcohol Program Manager and, except as provided below or by law, the results of any drug/alcohol test shall not be disclosed without express written consent of the tested employee.

    (1)   The employee, upon written request, is entitled to obtain copies of any records pertaining to their use of prohibited drugs or misuse of alcohol including any drug or alcohol testing records. Covered employees have the right to gain access to any pertinent records such as equipment calibration records, and records of laboratory certifications. Employees may not have access to SAP referrals and follow-up testing plans.

    (2)   Records of a verified positive drug/alcohol test result shall be released to the Drug and Alcohol Program Manager, Department Supervisor and Personnel Manager on a need to know basis.

    (3)   Records will be released to a subsequent employer only upon receipt of a written request from the employee.

    (4)   Records of an employee's drug/alcohol tests shall be released to the adjudicator in a grievance, lawsuit, or other proceeding initiated by or on behalf of the tested individual arising from the results of the drug/alcohol test. The records will be released to the decision maker in the preceding. The information will only be released with binding stipulation from the decision maker will make it available only to parties in the preceding.

    (5)   Records will be released to the National Transportation Safety Board during an accident investigation.

    (6)   Records will be released to the DOT or any DOT agency with regulatory authority over the employer or any of its employees.

    (7)   Records will be released if requested by a Federal, state or local safety agency with regulatory authority over _____ or the employee.

    (8)   If a party seeks a court order to release a specimen or part of a specimen contrary to any provision of Part 40 as amended necessary legal steps to contest the issuance of the order will be taken.

    (9)   In cases of a contractor or sub-recipient of a state department of transportation, records will be released when requested by such agencies that must certify compliance with the regulation to the FTA.

U. SYSTEM CONTACTS

Any questions regarding this policy or any other aspect of the substance abuse policy should be directed to the following individual(s):

_____ Drug and Alcohol Program Manager:

Name:
Title:
Address:
Telephone Number:

Medical Review Officer

Name:
Title:
Address:
Telephone Number:

Substance Abuse Professional

Name:
Title:
Address:
Telephone Number:

HHS Certified Laboratory Primary Specimen

Name:
Address:
Telephone Number:

HHS Certified Laboratory Split Specimen

Name:
Address:
Telephone Number:

This Policy was adopted by the _____

on _____,2002.

_____

Attachment A
Safety-Sensitive Positions

<u>—Administration Covered Classifications</u>

Title   **Testing Authority**

<u>— **Job Classifications**</u>

<u>Title</u>   <u>Testing Authority</u>

Attachment B
Alcohol Fact Sheet

Alcohol is a socially acceptable drug that has been consumed throughout the world for centuries. It is considered a recreational beverage when consumed in moderation for enjoyment and relaxation during social gatherings. However, when consumed primarily for its physical and mood-altering effects, it is a substance of abuse. As a depressant, it slows down physical responses and progressively impairs mental functions.

    Signs and Symptoms of Use

- Dulled mental processes
- Lack of coordination
- Odor of alcohol on breath
- Possible constricted pupils
- Sleepy or stupor us condition
- Slowed reaction rate
- Slurred speech

(Note: Except for the odor, these are general signs and symptoms of any depressant substance.)

☐ Health Effects

The chronic consumption of alcohol (average of three servings per day of beer [12 ounces], whiskey [1 ounce], or wine [6 ounce glass]) over time may result in the following health hazards:

- Decreased sexual functioning
- Dependency (up to 10 percent of all people who drink alcohol become physically and/or mentally dependent on alcohol and can be termed "alcoholic")
- Fatal liver diseases
- Increased cancers of the mouth, tongue, pharynx, esophagus, rectum, breast, and malignant melanoma
- Kidney disease
- Pancreatitis
- Spontaneous abortion and neonatal mortality
- Ulcers
- Birth defects (up to 54 percent of all birth defects are alcohol related).

☐ Social Issues

- Two-thirds of all homicides are committed by people who drink prior to the crime.
- Two to three percent of the driving population is legally drunk at any one time. This rate is doubled at night and on weekends.
- Two-thirds of all Americans will be involved in an alcohol-related vehicle accident during their lifetimes.
- The rate of separation and divorce in families with alcohol dependency problems is 7 times the average.
- Forty percent of family court cases are alcohol problem related.

. Alcoholics are 15 times more likely to commit suicide than are other segments of the population.

. More than 60 percent of burns, 40 percent of falls, 69 percent of boating accidents, and 76 percent of private aircraft accidents are alcohol related.

□ The Annual Toll

. 24,000 people will die on the highway due to the legally impaired driver.

. 12,000 more will die on the highway due to the alcohol-affected driver.

. 15,800 will die in non-highway accidents.

. 30,000 will die due to alcohol-caused liver disease.

. 10,000 will die due to alcohol-induced brain disease or suicide.

. Up to another 125,000 will die due to alcohol-related conditions or accidents.

□ Workplace Issues

. It takes one hour for the average person (150 pounds) to process one serving of an alcoholic beverage from the body.

. Impairment in coordination and judgment can be objectively measured with as little as two drinks in the body.

. A person who is legally intoxicated is 6 times more likely to have an accident than a sober person.

Attachment C
Minimum Thresholds

INITIAL TEST CUTOFF LEVELS
(ng/ml)

Marijuana metabolites	50
Cocaine metabolites	300
Opiate metabolites	2,000
Phencyclidine	25
Amphetamines	1,000

CONFIRMATORY TEST CUT/OFF LEVELS   (ng/ml)

Marijuana metabolites	15
Cocaine metabolites	150
Opiates:	
Morphine	2,000
Codeine	2,000
Phencyclidine	25
Amphetamines:	
Amphetamines	500
Methamphetamine	500

6. Georgia Department of Transportation

TABLE OF CONTENTS

<table>
<tr><td>

Georgia Department of Transportation
Fitness for Duty Policy
Drug and Alcohol Testing Program[1]

</td><td>

Insert date of last revision.

</td></tr>
</table>

Bold = FTA requirements
Italics = Drug-Free Workplace Act of 1988 requirements

1.0   POLICY

The __See Note 1__ is dedicated to providing safe, dependable, and economical transportation services to our transit system passengers. Transit system employees are our most valuable resource and it is our goal to provide a healthy, satisfying working environment which promotes personal opportunities for growth. In meeting these goals, it is our policy (1) to ensure that employees are not impaired in their ability to perform assigned duties in a safe, productive, and healthy manner; (2) to create a workplace environment free from the adverse effects of drug abuse and alcohol misuse; (3) to prohibit the unlawful manufacture, distribution, dispensing, possession, or use of controlled substances; and (4) to encourage employees to seek professional assistance anytime personal problems, including alcohol or drug dependency, adversely affect their ability to perform their assigned duties.

Note 1. Insert name of transit system.

2.0   PURPOSE

The purpose of this policy is to __See Note 2__. This policy is also intended to comply with all applicable Federal regulations governing workplace anti-drug and alcohol programs in the transit industry. The Federal Transit Administration (FTA) of the U.S. Department of Transportation has published 49 CFR Part 655 as amended, that mandate urine drug testing and breath alcohol testing for safety-sensitive positions and prohibits performance of safety-sensitive functions when there is a positive test result. The U.S. Department of Transportation (DOT) has also published 49 CFR Part 40, as amended, which sets standards for the collection and testing of urine and breath specimens. In addition, the Federal government published 49 CFR Part 29, "The Drug-Free Workplace Act of 1988," which requires the establishment of drug-free workplace policies and the reporting of certain drug-related offenses to the FTA. This policy incorporates those requirements for safety-sensitive employees and others when so noted.

Note 2. Insert discussion of purpose and objectives of your program, i.e., ensure worker fitness for duty and to protect our employees, passengers, and the public from the risks posed by the misuse of alcohol and use of prohibited drugs.

Note 3. List covered employees, i.e., safety-sensitive and/or non-safety-sensitive employees.

3.0   APPLICABILITY

This policy applies to all __See Note 3__ **and contractors** when they are on transit property or **when performing any transit-related safety-sensitive or** non-safety-sensitive **business**. This policy applies to off-site lunch periods or breaks when an employee is scheduled to return to work. **See Note 4** .

A safety-sensitive function is any duty related to the safe operation of mass transit service including the operation of a revenue service vehicle

Note 4. Expand applicability to reflect additional employees, time periods, etc. to which the policy will apply, i.e., visitors, vendors, and contractor employees are governed by this policy while on transit premises and will not be permitted to conduct transit business if found to violate this policy.

---

[1] **All provisions in bold face print are consistent with requirements in 49 CFR Part 655 or Part 40, as amended. Provisions in italics are set forth in the Drug-Free Workplace Act (49 CFR Part 29). All other provisions are set forth under the authority of the transit system.**

(whether or not the vehicle is in revenue service), dispatch, maintenance of a revenue service vehicle or equipment used in revenue service, security personnel who carry firearms, and any other employee who holds a Commercial Driver's License. Maintenance functions include the repair, overhaul, and rebuild of engines, vehicles and/or equipment. A list of safety-sensitive positions who perform one or more of the above mentioned duties is attached. See Note 5

> **Note 5. Attach list of safety-sensitive positions specific to your system.**

4.0   PROHIBITED SUBSTANCES

"Prohibited substances" addressed by this policy include the following:

4.1   Illegally Used Controlled Substances or Drugs

The use of any illegal drug or any substance identified in Schedules I through V of Section 202 of the Controlled Substance Act (21 U.S.C. 812), as further defined by 21 CFR 1300.11 through 1300.15 is prohibited at all times unless a legal prescription has been written for the substance. This includes, but is not limited to: marijuana, amphetamines, opiates, phencyclidine (PCP), and cocaine, as well as any drug not approved for medical use by the U.S. Drug Enforcement Administration or the U.S. Food and Drug Administration. Illegal use includes use of any illegal drug, misuse of legal prescribed drugs, and use of illegally obtained prescription drugs. **Safety-sensitive employees will be tested for marijuana, cocaine, amphetamines, opiates, and phencyclidine as described in Section 6.0 of this policy.**

4.2   Legal Drugs

 The appropriate use of legally prescribed drugs and non-prescription medications is not prohibited. _____**See Note 6**____.

A legally prescribed drug means that individual has a prescription or other written approval from a physician for the use of a drug in the course of medical treatment. It must include the patient's name, the name of the substance, quantity/amount to be taken, and the period of authorization. The misuse or abuse of legal drugs while performing transit business is prohibited.

Also the use of medical marijuana and hemp products which present levels of drugs or drug metabolites above the DOT minimum thresholds, is considered a violation of this policy.

4.3   Alcohol

The use of beverages containing alcohol or substances including any medication, mouthwash, food, candy, or any other substance such that alcohol is present in the body while performing transit business is prohibited. The concentration of alcohol is expressed in terms of alcohol per 210 liters of breath as measured by an evidential breath testing device.

> **Note 6. Describe local policy on the prohibition of legal drugs and performance-altering prescription drugs** i.e., However, the use of any substance which carries a warning label that indicates that mental functioning, motor skills, or judgment may be adversely affected must be reported to supervisory personnel and medical advice and written authorization from the attending physician must be sought by the employee, as appropriate, before performing work-related duties.

5.0 PROHIBITED CONDUCT

5.1 Manufacture, Trafficking, Possession, and Use

Transit system employees are prohibited from engaging in the unlawful manufacture, distribution, dispensing, possession, or use of prohibited substances on transit authority premises, in transit vehicles, in uniform or while on *transit authority business.* Employees who violate this provision will be subject to ____**See Note 7**___. Law enforcement shall be notified, as appropriate, where criminal activity is suspected.

> *Note 7. Insert transit system discipline*

5.2 Intoxication/Under the Influence

Any ___**See Note 8**_____ employee who is reasonable suspected of being intoxicated, impaired, under the influence of a prohibited substance, or not fit for duty shall be suspended from job duties pending an investigation and verification of condition. Employees found to be under the influence of a prohibited substance or **who fail to pass a drug or alcohol test shall be removed from duty** and ____**See Note 9**_. **A drug or alcohol test is considered positive if the individual is found to have a quantifiable presence of a prohibited substance in the body above the minimum thresholds defined in 49 CFR Part 40, as amended.**

> *Note 8. List covered employees,* i.e., safety-sensitive and/or non-safety-sensitive.

> *Note 9. Insert transit system discipline.*

5.3 Alcohol and Drug Use

No **See Note 10** **employee should report for duty or remain on duty when his/her ability to perform assigned safety-sensitive functions is adversely affected by alcohol or when his/her breath alcohol concentration is 0.04 or greater.** No ___**See Note 10**___**employee shall use alcohol** while on duty, in uniform, **while performing safety-sensitive functions, or just before or just after performing a safety-sensitive function. No ____See Note 10____ employee shall use alcohol within four hours of reporting for duty, or during the hours that they are on call.**

> *Note 10. List covered employees,* i.e., safety-sensitive and/or non-safety-sensitive.

All safety sensitive employees are prohibited from reporting for duty or remaining on duty any time there is a quantifiable presence of a prohibited substance in the body above the minimum thresholds defined in 49 CFR Part 40, as amended. Violation of these provisions is prohibited and punishable ____**See Note 11**_____.

> *Note 11. Insert transit system discipline.*

5.4 Compliance with Testing Requirements

All _____See Note 12_____ employees will be subject to urine drug testing and breath alcohol testing as a condition of employment. Any See Note 12_____ **employee who refuses to comply with a request for testing shall be removed from duty and _____See Note 13_____.** **Any ____See Note 12_____ employee who is suspected of providing false information in connection with a test, or who is suspected of falsifying test results through tampering, contamination, adulteration, or substitution will be required to undergo an observed collection. Verification of falsifying test results will result in** See Note 13_____ **The following are also considered a refusal to test if the employee:**

> *Note 12. List covered employees,* i.e., safety-sensitive and/or non-safety-sensitive.

> *Note 13. Insert transit system discipline.*

- Fails to appear for any test within a reasonable time, as determined by the employer, after being directed to do so by the employer
- Fails to remain at the testing site until the testing process is complete
- Fails to provide a urine or breath specimen for any drug test required by this part or DOT agency regulations
- In the case of a directly observed or monitored collection in a drug test, fails to permit the observation or monitoring of your provision of a specimen
- Fails to provide a sufficient amount of urine or breath when directed, and it has been determined, through a required medical evaluation, that there was no adequate medical explanation for the failure
- Fails or declines to take a second test the employer or collector has directed you to take;
- Fails to undergo a medical examination or evaluation, as directed by the MRO as part of the verification process, or as directed by the DER as part of the "shy bladder"' or "shy lung" procedures
- Fails to cooperate with any part of the testing process (e.g., refuse to empty pockets when so directed by the collector, behave in a confrontational way that disrupts the collection process).
- If the MRO reports that there is verified adulterated or substituted test result,

Drug tests can be performed any time a safety-sensitive employee is on duty. An alcohol test can be performed when the safety sensitive employee is actually performing a safety-sensitive duty, just before, or just after the performance of a safety-sensitive duty.

5.5   Treatment Requirements   _____See Note 14_____

All employees are encouraged to make use of the available resources for treatment for alcohol misuse and illegal drug use problems. Under certain circumstances, employees may be required to undergo treatment for substance abuse or alcohol misuse. Any employee who refuses or fails to comply with transit system requirements for treatment, after care, or return to duty shall be subject to disciplinary action, up to and including termination. The cost of any treatment or rehabilitation services will be paid for directly by the employee or their insurance provider. Employees will be allowed to take accumulated sick leave and vacation leave to participate in the prescribed rehabilitation program.

> *Note 14. Section 5.5 is optional. If included, reflect local situation for treatment, self-referrals, management referrals, who pays, and potential use of leave.*

5.6   Notifying the Transit System of Criminal Drug Conviction

All employees are required to notify the transit system of any criminal drug statute conviction for a violation occurring in the workplace within five days after such conviction. Failure to comply with this provision shall result in _____**See Note 15**_____.

> *Note 15. Insert transit system discipline.*

5.7   Proper Application of the Policy   _____See Note 16_____

The transit system is dedicated to assuring fair and equitable application of this substance abuse policy. Therefore, supervisors/managers are required to use and apply all aspects of this policy in an unbiased and impartial manner. Any supervisor/manager who knowingly disregards the requirements of this policy, or who is found to deliberately misuse the policy in regard to subordinates, shall be subject to disciplinary action in accordance with the provisions set forth in the personnel manual.

> *Note 16. Section 5.7 is optional. If included, state the local decision as to manager/supervisor responsibility and subsequent discipline.*

6.0   TESTING PROCEDURES

Analytical urine drug testing and breath testing for alcohol may be conducted when circumstance warrant or as required by Federal regulations. All **See Note 17** **employees shall be subject to drug testing prior to employment, for reasonable suspicion, and following an accident as defined in Section 6.2, 6.3, and 6.4 of this policy. All   See Note 17   employees shall be subject to alcohol testing for reasonable suspicion and following an accident as defined in Section 6.2, 6.3, and 6.4. In addition, all   See Note 17   employees will be tested prior to returning to duty after failing a drug or alcohol test and after completion of the Substance Abuse Professional's recommended treatment program and subsequent release to duty. Follow-up testing will also be conducted following return to duty for a period of one to five years, with at least six tests performed during the first year.**

> *Note 17. List covered employees,* i.e., safety-sensitive and/or non-safety-sensitive.

Those employees who perform safety-sensitive functions as defined in the Attachment 1 shall also be subject to testing on a random, unannounced basis.

Testing shall be conducted in a manner to assure a high degree of accuracy and reliability and using techniques, equipment, and laboratory facilities which have been approved by the U.S. Department of Health and Human Service (DHHS). All testing will be conducted consistent with the procedures put forth in 49 CFR Part 40, as amended. The procedures will be performed in a private, confidential manner and every effort will be made to protect the employee, the integrity of the drug testing procedure, and the validity of the test result.

The drugs that will be tested for include marijuana, cocaine, opiates, amphetamines, and phencyclidine. Urine specimens will be collected using the split specimen collection method described in 49 CFR Part 40. Each specimen will be accompanied by a DOT Chain of Custody and Control Form and identified using a unique identification number that attributes the specimen to the correct individual. An initial drug screen will be conducted on the primary urine specimen. For those specimens that are not negative, appear to be substitute, or adulterated, a confirmatory Gas Chromatography/Mass Spectrometry (GC/MS) test will be performed. The test will be considered positive if the amounts present are above the minimum thresholds established in 49 CFR Part 40, as amended. Attachment 3 lists the minimum thresholds established for each drug and/or its metabolites.   The test results from the laboratory will be reported to a Medical Review Officer. A Medical Review Officer (MRO) is a licensed physician with detailed knowledge of substance abuse disorders and drug testing. The MRO will review the test results to ensure the scientific validity of the test and to determine whether there is a legitimate medical explanation for a confirmed positive test result, substitution or adulteration. The MRO will contact the employee, notify the employee of the positive, substitute, or adulterated laboratory result, and provide the employee with an opportunity to explain the confirmed test result. The MRO will subsequently review the employee's medical history/medical records to determine whether there is a legitimate medical explanation for a positive, substitute or adulterated laboratory result. If no legitimate medical explanation is found, the test will be verified positive, substitute, or adulterated and reported to the company program manager. If a legitimate explanation is found, the MRO will report the test result as negative.

The split specimen will be stored at the initial laboratory until the analysis of the primary specimen is completed. If the primary specimen is negative, the split will be discarded. If the primary is

---

positive, the split will be retained for testing if so requested by the employee through the Medical Review Officer. See Note 18

Observed collections:

Consistent with 49 CFR part 40 collection under direct observation (by a person of the same gender) with no advance notice will occur if:

(1) The laboratory reports to the MRO that a specimen is invalid, and the MRO reports to _____ that there was not an adequate medical explanation for the result; or

(2) The MRO reports to _____ that the original positive, adulterated, or substituted test result had to be cancelled because the test of the split specimen could not be performed.

   (a) _____ may direct a collection under direct observation of an employee if the drug test is a return-to-duty test or a follow-up test.

   (b) The collector, must immediately conduct a collection under direct observation if:

They are directed by _____ to do so; or

(3) The collector observes materials brought to the collection site or the employee's conduct clearly indicates an attempt to tamper with a specimen; or

   (4) The temperature on the original specimen was out of range; or

   (5) The original specimen appeared to have been tampered with.

> Note 18. *Indicate if you want to test for additional drugs, or if you want to reserve the right to,* i.e., in instances where there is a reason to believe an employee is abusing a substance other that the five drugs listed above, the transit system reserves the right to test for additional drugs under the transit system's own authority using standard laboratory testing protocols.

Tests for breath alcohol concentration will be conducted utilizing a National Highway Traffic Safety Administration (NHTSA)-approved testing device operated by a trained technician. If the initial test indicates an alcohol concentration of 0.02 or greater, a second test will be performed to confirm the results of the initial test. The confirmatory test will be performed using a NHTSA-approved evidential breath testing device (EBT) operated by a trained breath alcohol technician (BAT). The EBT will identify each test by a unique sequential identification number. This number, time, and unit identifier will be provided on each EBT printout. The EBT printout along with an approved alcohol testing form will be used to document the test, the subsequent results, and to attribute the test to the correct employee. The test will be performed in a private, confidential manner as required by 49 CFR Part 40 as amended. The procedure will be followed as prescribed to protect the employee and to maintain the integrity of the alcohol testing procedures and validity of the test result.

A See Note 19 employee who has a confirmed alcohol concentration of greater than 0.02 but less than 0.04 will be removed from his/her position for eight hours unless a retest results in a concentration measure of less than 0.02. See Note 20 An alcohol concentration of 0.04 or greater will be considered a positive alcohol test and in violation of this policy and a violation of the requirements set forth in 49 CFR Part 655 for safety-sensitive employees.

Any See Note 21 employee that has a confirmed positive drug or alcohol test will be removed from his/her position, informed of educational and rehabilitation programs available, and referred to a Substance Abuse Professional (SAP) for assessment. A positive drug and/or alcohol test will also result in See Note 22 .

> Note 19. *List covered employees,* i.e., safety-sensitive and/or non-safety-sensitive.

> Note 20. *Insert consequences for alcohol test results of 0.02 - 0.039.*

> Note 21. *List covered employees,* i.e., safety-sensitive and/or non-safety-sensitive.

> Note 22. *Insert transit discipline.*

6.1 Employee Requested Testing

Any ___See Note 23___ employee who questions the results of a required drug test under paragraphs 6.2 through 6.7 of this policy may request that the split sample be tested. This test must be conducted at a different DHHS-certified laboratory. The test must be conducted on the split sample that was provided by the employee at the same time as the original sample. ___See Note 24___. The method of collecting, storing, and testing the split sample will be consistent with the procedures set forth in 49 CFR Part 40, as amended. The employee's request for a split sample test must be made to the Medical Review Officer within 72 hours of notice of the original sample verified test result. Requests after 72 hours will only be accepted if the delay was due to documentable facts that were beyond the control of the employee.

> *Note 23. List covered employees,* i.e., safety-sensitive and/or non-safety-sensitive.

> *Note 24. Indicate that the split sample test will occur regardless of up-front payment, but that the transit system reserves the right to seek reimbursement from the employee.*

6.2 Pre-Employment Testing

All___See Note 25___ position applicants shall undergo urine drug testing prior to hire or transfer into a safety-sensitive position. Receipt by the transit system of a negative drug test result is required prior to employment. Failure of a pre-employment drug test will disqualify an applicant for employment for a period of___See Note 26. **Evidence of the absence of drug dependency from a Substance Abuse Professional that meets with the approval of the DOT and negative pre-employment drug tests will be required prior to further consideration for employment.** The cost for assessment and any subsequent treatment will be for the sole responsibility of the individual.

> *Note 25. List covered employees,* i.e., safety-sensitive and/or non-safety-sensitive.

> *Note 26. Insert period of disqualification and re-application process.*

In addition, FTA requires all safety sensitive employees who have been off duty for 90 or more days for any reason are required to successfully pass a pre-employment drug test prior to the performance of a safety-sensitive function.

A pre-employment/pre-transfer test will also be performed anytime an employee's status changes from an inactive status in a safety-sensitive position to an active status in a safety-sensitive position (i.e., return from Worker's Comp., return from leave of absence).

6.3 Reasonable Suspicion Testing

All See Note 27___ employees may be subject to a fitness for duty evaluation, and **urine and/or breath testing when there are reasons to believe that drug or alcohol use is adversely affecting job performance. A reasonable suspicion referral for testing will be made on the basis of documented objective facts and circumstances which are consistent with the short-term effects of substance abuse or alcohol misuse.** Examples of reasonable suspicion include, but are not limited to, the following:

> *Note 27. List covered employees,* i.e., safety-sensitive and/or non-safety-sensitive.

1. Physical signs and symptoms consistent with prohibited substance use or alcohol misuse.
2. Evidence of the manufacture, distribution, dispensing, possession, or use of controlled substances, drugs, alcohol, or other prohibited substance.
3. Occurrence of a serious or potentially serious accident that may have been caused by prohibited substance abuse or alcohol misuse.
4. Fights (to mean physical contact), assaults, and flagrant disregard or violations of established safety, security, or other operating procedures

Reasonable suspicion referrals must be made by a supervisor who is trained to detect the signs and symptoms of drug and alcohol use and who reasonably concludes that an employee may be adversely affected or impaired in his/her work performance due to possible prohibited substance abuse or alcohol misuse.

6.4   Post-Accident Testing

All safety-sensitive employees will be required to undergo urine and breath testing if they are involved in an accident with a _____ Transit vehicle (regardless of whether or not the vehicle is in revenue service) that results in a fatality. This includes all surviving safety-sensitive employees that operated the vehicle and any other whose performance could have contributed to the accident. In addition, a post-accident test will be conducted if an accident results in injuries requiring immediate transportation to a medical treatment facility or one or more vehicles incurs disabling damage, unless the operator can be completely discounted as a contributing factor to the accident. The accident definition may include some incidents where an individual is injured even though there is no vehicle collision.

Following an accident, the safety-sensitive employees will be tested as soon as possible, but no to exceed eight hours for alcohol testing and 32 hours for drug testing. Any safety-sensitive employee involved in an accident must refrain from alcohol use for eight hours following the accident or until he/she undergoes a post-accident alcohol test. Any safety-sensitive employee who leaves the scene of the accident without justifiable explanation prior to submission to drug and alcohol testing will be considered to have refused the test _____ See Note 28 _____. Employees tested under this provision will include not only the operations personnel, but any other covered employee whose performance could have contributed to the accident.

> *Note 28. Insert transit system discipline.*

If the Transit system is unable to perform a FTA drug and alcohol test (i.e., employee is unconscious, employee is detained by law enforcement agency), the transit system may use drug and alcohol post-accident test results administered by State and local law enforcement officials. The State and local law enforcement officials must have independent authority for the test and the employer must obtain the results in conformance with state and local law.

6.5   Random Testing

Employees in safety-sensitive positions will be subjected to random, unannounced testing. The selection of safety-sensitive employees for random drug and alcohol testing will be made using a scientifically valid method that ensures each covered employee that they will have an equal chance of being selected each time selections are made. The random tests will be unannounced and spread throughout the year. Tests can be conducted at any time during an employee's shift (i.e. beginning, middle, end). Employees are required to proceed immediately to the collection site upon notification of their random selection.

6.6   Return-To-Duty Testing

All _____ See Note 29 _____ employees who tested positive on a drug or alcohol test will be _____ See Note 30 _____. However, in the event an employee returns to duty, he/she must test negative on both a return-to-duty test and a drug and alcohol test (below 0.02 for alcohol) and be evaluated and released to duty by the Substance Abuse Professional before returning to work. A Substance

> *Note 29. List covered employees, i.e., safety-sensitive and/or non-safety-sensitive.*
>
> *Note 30. Insert employee discipline.*

Abuse Professional (SAP) is a licensed physician or certified psychologist, social worker, employee assistance professional, or addiction counselor certified by the National Association of Alcoholism and Drug Abuse Counselors Certification Commission or by the International Certification Reciprocity Consortium/Alcohol and Other Drug Abuse. The SAP must also have clinical experience in the diagnosis and treatment of drug and alcohol related diseases. Before scheduling the return to duty test, the SAP must assess the employee and determine if the required treatment has been completed.

6.7 Follow-Up Testing

_____See Note 31_____ employees will be required to undergo frequent unannounced urine and/or breath testing following their return to duty. The follow-up testing will be performed for a period of one to five years with a minimum of six tests to be performed the first year. The frequency and duration of the follow-up tests beyond the minimum will be determined by a qualified Substance Abuse Professional.

Note 31. List covered employees, i.e., safety-sensitive and/or non-safety-sensitive.

7.0   EMPLOYMENT ASSESSMENT   See Note 32

Note 32. Modify to reflect local decisions on assessment, EAPs, and treatment.

Any ___See Note 33___ employee who tests positive for the presence of illegal drugs or alcohol above the minimum thresholds set forth in 49 CFR Part 40, as amended, will be referred for evaluation by a Substance Abuse Professional (SAP). A SAP is a licensed or certified physician, psychologist, social worker, employee assistance profession, or addiction counselor with knowledge of and clinical experience in the diagnosis and treatment of alcohol and drug-related disorders. If the employee is eligible for a second chance, a SAP will evaluate him/her to determine what assistance is needed to resolve problems associated with prohibited drug use or alcohol misuse.

Note 33. List covered employees, i.e., safety-sensitive and/or non-safety-sensitive.

Assessment by a SAP_____See Note 34___ does not shield an employee from disciplinary action or guarantee employment or reinstatement with the transit system. The ___See Note 35___ should be consulted to determine the penalty for performance-based infractions and violation of policy provisions.

Note 34. Refer to employee assistance program if you have one in place.

Note 35. Refer to transit system's disciplinary code.

If a ___See Note 36___ employee is allowed to return -to-duty, he/she must properly follow the rehabilitation program prescribed by the SAP, the employee must have negative return-to-duty drug and alcohol tests, and be subject to unannounced follow-up testing for a period of one to five years. ___See Note 37___ .

Note 36. List covered employees, i.e., safety-sensitive and/or non-safety-sensitive.

Note 37. Who will pay for treatment and rehabilitation services and will time off be granted, i.e., the cost of any treatment or rehabilitation services will be paid directly by the employee or the insurance provider. Employees will be allowed to take accumulated sick leave and vacation leave to participate in prescribed rehabilitation program.

8.0   INFORMATION DISCLOSURE

To be considered for employment, all applicants will be asked to give consent to (Insert Transit System Name) for a background check of their previous DOT covered employer over the past two years. Information requested will include:
1. Alcohol test results of 0.04 or higher alcohol concentration.
2. Verified positive drug tests.
3. Refusals to be tested (including verified adulterated or substituted drug test results.)

4. Other violations of DOT agency drug and alcohol testing regulations.

5. With respect to any employee who violated a DOT drug and alcohol regulation, documentation of the employee's successful completion of DOT return-to-duty requirements (including follow-up tests).

All drug and alcohol testing records will be maintained in a secure manner so that disclosure of information to unauthorized persons does not occur. Information will only be released in the following circumstances:

1. To a third party only as directed by specific, written instruction of the employee

2. To the decision-maker in a lawsuit, grievance, or other proceeding initiated by or on the behalf of the employee tested

3. To a subsequent employer upon receipt of a written request from the employee

4. To the National Transportation Safety Board during an accident investigation

5. To the DOT or any DOT agency with regulatory authority over the employer or any of its employees, or to a State oversight agency authorized to oversee rail fixed-guideway systems

6. To the employee, upon written request

7. Records will be released if requested by a Federal, state or local safety agency with regulatory authority over _____ or the employee.

8. If a party seeks a court order to release a specimen or part of a specimen contrary to any provision of Part 40 necessary legal steps to contest the issuance of the order will be taken.

9.0 EMPLOYEE AND SUPERVISOR TRAINING

All safety sensitive employees will undergo a minimum of 60 minutes of training on the signs and symptoms of drug use including the effects and consequences of drug use on personal health, safety, and the work environment. The training must also include manifestations and behavioral cues that may indicate prohibited drug use.

Supervisors will also receive 60 minutes of reasonable suspicion training on the physical, behavioral, and performance indicators of probable drug use and 60 minutes of additional reasonable suspicion training on the physical, behavioral, speech, and performance indicators of probable alcohol misuse.

Information on the signs, symptoms, health affects and consequences of alcohol misuse is presented in Attachment 2.

10.0 RE-ENTRY CONTRACTS   See Note 38

Employees who re-enter the workforce must agree to a re-entry contract. That contract may include (but is not limited to):

1. A release to work statement from the Substance Abuse Professional.

2. A negative test for drugs and/or alcohol.

3. An agreement to unannounced frequent follow-up testing for a period of one to five years with at least six tests performed the first year.

4. A statement of work-related behaviors.

5. An agreement to follow specified after care requirements with the understanding that violation of the re-entry contract is grounds for termination.

Note 38. Include Section 10.0 only if you allow employees to return to duty and you require re-entry contracts. Be sure the items listed reflect the items typically included in your re-entry contracts. If you do not use re-entry contracts, this portion of the policy should be omitted.

11.0   SYSTEM CONTACT

Any questions regarding this policy or any other aspect of the drug free and alcohol-free transit program should contact the following transit system representative:

Program Manager:

Name: _____See Note 39_____
Title:
Address:
Telephone Number:
FAX Number:

> *Note 39. Insert name and address of program manager.*

Medical Review Officer :

Name: _____See Note 40_____
Address:
Telephone Number:
FAX Number:

> *Note 40. Insert name and address of medical review officer.*

Substance Abuse Professional :

Name: _____See Note 41_____
Title:
Address:
Telephone Number:
FAX Number:

> *Note 41. Insert name and address of substance abuse professional.*

Attachment 1
Safety-Sensitive and Non-Safety-Sensitive Functions

Every transit system employee should be included on one of the following lists. You must be able to defend why each position is placed in its respective lists:

Safety-Sensitive Functions

> List specific job titles of those who perform safety-sensitive job functions.

Non-Safety-Sensitive Functions

> List specific job titles of those who do not perform safety-sensitive job functions.

Attachment 2
Alcohol Fact Sheet

Alcohol is a socially acceptable drug that has been consumed throughout the world for centuries. It is considered a recreational beverage when consumed in moderation for enjoyment and relaxation during social gatherings. However, when consumed primarily for its physical and mood-altering effects, it is a substance of abuse. As a depressant, it slows down physical responses and progressively impairs mental functions.

Signs and Symptoms of Use

- Dulled mental processes
- Lack of coordination
- Odor of alcohol on breath
- Possible constricted pupils
- Sleepy or stuporous condition
- Slowed reaction rate
- Slurred speech

(Note: Except for the odor, these are general signs and symptoms of any depressant substance.)

Health Effects

The chronic consumption of alcohol (average of three servings per day of beer [12 ounces], whiskey [1 ounce], or wine [6 ounce glass]) over time may result in the following health hazards:

- Decreased sexual functioning

- Dependency (up to 10 percent of all people who drink alcohol become physically and/or mentally dependent on alcohol and can be termed "alcoholic")

- Fatal liver diseases

- Increased cancers of the mouth, tongue, pharynx, esophagus, rectum, breast, and malignant melanoma

- Kidney disease

- Pancreatitis

- Spontaneous abortion and neonatal mortality

- Ulcers

- Birth defects (up to 54 percent of all birth defects are alcohol related).

Social Issues

♦ Two-thirds of all homicides are committed by people who drink prior to the crime.

♦ Two to three percent of the driving population is legally drunk at any one time. This rate is doubled at night and on weekends.

♦ Two-thirds of all Americans will be involved in an alcohol-related vehicle accident during their lifetimes.

♦ The rate of separation and divorce in families with alcohol dependency problems is 7 times the average.

♦ Forty percent of family court cases are alcohol problem related.

♦ Alcoholics are 15 times more likely to commit suicide than are other segments of the population.

♦ More than 60 percent of burns, 40 percent of falls, 69 percent of boating accidents, and 76 percent of private aircraft accidents are alcohol related.

The Annual Toll

♦ 24,000 people will die on the highway due to the legally impaired driver.
♦ 12,000 more will die on the highway due to the alcohol-affected driver.
♦ 15,800 will die in non-highway accidents.
♦ 30,000 will die due to alcohol-caused liver disease.
♦ 10,000 will die due to alcohol-induced brain disease or suicide.
♦ Up to another 125,000 will die due to alcohol-related conditions or accidents.

Workplace Issues

♦ It takes one hour for the average person (150 pounds) to process one serving of an alcoholic beverage from the body.

♦ Impairment in coordination and judgment can be objectively measured with as little as two drinks in the body.

♦ A person who is legally intoxicated is 6 times more likely to have an accident than a sober person.

Attachment 3
Minimum Thresholds

Initial Test	Initial test cutoff levels
Marijuana metabolites	50 ng/ml
Cocaine metabolites	300 ng/ml
Opiate metabolites	2,000 ng/ml
Phencyclidine (PCP)	25 ng/ml
Amphetamines	1,000 ng/ml

Confirmatory Test	Confirmatory test cutoff levels
Marijuana metabolites (1)	15 ng/ml
Cocaine metabolites (2)	150 ng/ml
Opiates:	
Morphine	2,000 ng/ml
Codeine	2,000 ng/ml
Phencyclidine (PCP)	25 ng/ml
Amphetamines:	
Amphetamine	500 ng/ml
Methamphetamine (3)	500 ng/ml

(1) Delta-9-tetrahydrocannabinol-9-carboxlic acid
(2) Benzoylecgonine
(3) Specimen must also contain amphetamine at a concentration greater than or equal to 200 ng/ml.

These cutoff levels are subject to change by the Department of Health and Human Services as advances in technology or other considerations warrant identification of these substances at other concentrations.

Appendix B. Example Administrative Forms and Lists

This appendix contains best practice examples of forms and lists that have been used successfully to assist with general administrative issues and concerns and the issues related to each of the four types of testing required for all employers: pre-employment, reasonable suspicion, post accident, and random. Each of these examples is referenced and described in Section 4.1. The examples appear in the following figures, by the aforementioned groups:

General Administrative Duties

B-1. MBTA Employee Certification of Receipt of Policy

B-2. WMATA Employee Certification of Receipt of Policy

B-3. Tri-Met Employee Certification of Receipt of Policy

B-4. Log of Covered Employees who Complete Substance Abuse Training

B-5. Log of Employees who Complete Reasonable Suspicion Training

B-6. Certificate for Completion of Reasonable Suspicion Training

B-7. Roles and Responsibilities of Department Substance Abuse Program Manager

B-8. Roles and Responsibilities of Department Program Coordinator

B-9. Roles and Responsibilities of Departmental Divisional Contacts

B-10. Roles and Responsibilities of Front-Line Supervisors

B-11. Drug and Alcohol Testing Log

B-12. Drug Test Result Summary Form

B-13. Supervisor Log for Drug and Alcohol Testing

B-14. Order for Testing

B-15. Notification of Testing

B-16. Notice of Positive Drug Test

B-17. Notice of Positive Alcohol Test

B-18. Employee Notification of Positive Test Result

B-19. Supervisor Notification of Positive Test Result

Pre-Employment Testing

B-20. Flow Chart for Pre-Employment Testing Process

B-21. Pre-Employment Documentation Summary Sheet

B-22. Pre-Employment Test Tracking Log

B-23. Applicant Notification of Positive Test Result

GENERAL ADMINISTRATIVE DUTIES

Figure B-1. MBTA Employee Certification of Receipt of Policy

MASSACHUSETTS BAY TRANSPORTATION AUTHORITY
DRUG AND ALCOHOL POLICY
VERIFICATION OF EMPLOYEE NOTICE

I have received a copy of the August 1, 2001 Massachusetts Bay Transportation Authority Drug and Alcohol Policy which outlines the rights, duties, and responsibilities of the Massachusetts Bay Transportation Authority and all employees of the Massachusetts Bay Transportation Authority.

_____   _____

Employee Number   **Area**   **Department**

_____   _____

Class Number   **Class Title**

_____

Name

_____

Employee Signature   **Date**

_____

MBTA Witness Signature   **Date**

Figure B-2. WMATA Employee Certification of Receipt of Policy

Washington Metropolitan Area Transit Authority

Certification Statement

Drug and Alcohol Testing Program

I have received a copy of the Policy Instruction, P/I 7.21/2 Drug and Alcohol Testing, and a copy of the Substance Abuse Policy and Employee Assistance Program. I understand that it is my responsibility to read and abide by the rules contained in these Policies.

_____   _____
Signature   Date

_____
Print Name

_____
Employee Number

Figure B-3. Tri-Met Employee Certification of Receipt of Policy[1]

TRI-MET DRUG & ALCOHOL ABUSE PROGRAM

Yes, I have received Tri-Met's packet of information containing a copy of the revised drug and alcohol policy, EAP brochure, and Question & Answer information.

Name:_____

Employee No.:_____

Signature:_____ Date: _____

---

[1] Tri-County Metropolitan Transit District, Portland, Oregon

Figure B-4. Log of Covered Employees who Complete Substance Abuse Training[2]

DRUG AND ALCOHOL TRAINING FOR COVERED EMPLOYEES

I certify that I have received 60 minutes of training on the effects and consequences of alcohol misuse and prohibited drug use on health, safety, personal life, and the work environment, and on the signs and symptoms which may indicate such use in accordance with Title 49 CFR § 655.14 (b) (1).

NAME	DEPARTMENT	DATE

_____   _____

INSTRUCTOR   **DATE**

---

[2] Cincinnati Metro

Figure B-5. Log of Employees who Complete Reasonable Suspicion Training[3]

REASONABLE SUSPICION TRAINING FOR SUPERVISORY EMPLOYEES

I certify that I have received 60 minutes of training describing the physical, behavioral, speech and performance indicators of alcohol misuse and 60 minutes of training on the performance indicators of probable drug use constituting the grounds for a reasonable suspicion test in with Title 49 CFR § 655.14 (b) (2).

NAME	DEPARTMENT	DATE

INSTRUCTOR   **DATE**

[3] Cincinnati Metro

Figure B-6. Certificate for Completion of Supervisor Training[4]

The Government of The Virgin Islands

Certifies That

_____

Supervisor

Has completed Supervisor Reasonable Suspicion Training for Drug Use and Alcohol Misuse in Accordance with 49 CFR Part 655

On _____ *(date)*

_____

Instructor

[4] The Government of The Virgin Islands

Figure B-7. Roles and Responsibilities of Department Substance Abuse Program Manager [5]

ROLES AND RESPONSIBILITIES: SUBSTANCE ABUSE PROGRAM MANAGER

— Directs and manages the City's Substance Abuse program

— Supervises the City's Substance Abuse Program staff including the City personnel that perform the following:
- Random number pool management and selection
- Substance abuse professional services

— Manages, monitors, and enforces contracts for testing services, including:
- Collection sites
  ⇒ Urine specimen collection
  ⇒ Breath specimen collection (BATs)
- SED testing laboratory
- Split specimen laboratory
- Medical Review Officer

— Performs quality control checks on testing services:
- Mock audits
- Blind sample quality control checks
- Periodic inspections
- Review policies/procedures, checklists for being complete, up-to-date, and compliant with 49CFR Part 40
- Monitor/investigate employee complaints
- Periodic assessment of service provider credentials

— Maintains a thorough, current knowledge of all Federal drug and alcohol testing regulations including testing procedures (49CFR Part 40); FTA regulations (49CFR Part 655); and FHWA regulations (49CFR Part 382).

— Maintain a thorough and current knowledge of all other Federal, State, and Municipal legislation, regulations and case law regarding substance abuse testing that may pertain to City employee.

— Maintain a thorough and current knowledge of testing procedures, protocols, adulterants, and other relevant issues relating to drug and alcohol testing.

— Assist Department Program Coordinators with the successful, compliant, implementation of the City's Substance Abuse Policy.

— Advise Department Program Coordinators as they implement the program including policy implementation, discipline, and other issues as they arise.

— Recommend modifications to the City's Substance Abuse Policy as appropriate to reflect changes in regulations, operating environments, practical experience, and program administration. Present recommendations to the CAO and City Council, as appropriate.

— Develop training modules to train supervisors and other City employees on the City's policy and testing procedures.

— Coordinate training activities for/between City departments for supervisory Reasonable Suspicion and Drug Abuse/Alcohol misuse awareness training.

— Maintain a computerized database of testing records to facilitate the preparation/submission of MIS report required by Federal regulations.

— Maintain manual paper files to facilitate response to employee actions, lawsuits, grievances, audits, or other proceedings.

— Ensure confidentiality and security of all drug and alcohol testing records.

— Testify as necessary regarding the testing procedures and policies in administrative grievance procedures and lawsuits.

— Perform other duties as directed.

---

[5] City of Albuquerque

Figure B-8. Roles and Responsibilities of Department Program Coordinator[6]

ROLES AND RESPONSIBILITIES
DEPARTMENT PROGRAM COORDINATOR

— Coordinates with SAPM on program implementation.

— Responsible for policy implementation in department.

— Knowledgeable of regulatory compliance requirements as appropriate (Transit mandatory).

— Schedules random tests and works with Division Contact to ensure tests are performed.

— Re-schedules test in testing period if employee is unavailable on the testing day.

— Approves legitimate excuses for no test; takes corrective action when explanation is not legitimate.

— Notifies Random Selector when tests are not completed in the testing period.

— Tracks tests for department.

— Ensures that employees are properly coded as safety-sensitive or not.

— Works with Division Contacts to ensure that testing is performed within the regulatory guidelines –
   - Alcohol test only performed just before, during, just after the performance of a safety-sensitive job function
   - Drug test any time the covered employee is on duty
   - Tests performed as soon as possible following employee notification, accident, or reasonable suspicion determination
   - Document test delays of greater than 2 hours; discontinue alcohol test attempts after 8 hours; discontinue drug test attempt after 32 hours.

— Investigate procedural violations and take corrective actions as necessary

— Ensure appropriate department level documentation is completed accurately and in a timely manner; take corrective action as necessary.

— Maintain departmental records in a secure location.

— Schedule return-to-duty, and follow-up test consistent with SAP recommendation.

— Notify employees and department of positive test results; remove employee from duty; notify and refer to department for discipline; refer to SAP.

— Coordinate with SAP regarding employee's progress and return-to-duty status.

— Coordinate with SAPM regarding preparation and submission of annual MIS reports.

— Provide input to SAPM regarding quality of testing services; bring issues or problems to immediate attention of SAPM.

---

[6] City of Albuquerque

Figure B-9. Roles and Responsibilities of Departmental Divisional Contacts[7]

ROLES AND RESPONSIBILITIES
DEPARTMENTAL – DIVISION CONTACTS

— Upon notification of employees to be tested – check to make sure available on tests date. If not, inform DPC of need for alternate test date within testing period

— Arrange for employee to be removed from duty (schedule substitute as necessary), and notify of need for test

— Arrange for immediate transportation to collection site

— Notify DPC of post-accident and reasonable suspicion tests

— Ensure tests are complete consistent with regulatory requirements

— Ensure that all necessary documentation is complete and submitted to the DPC within 24 hours of the incident

Figure B-10. Roles and Responsibilities of Front-Line Supervisors [8]

ROLES AND RESPONSIBILITIES
FRONT-LINE SUPERVISORS

— Determine employee fitness for duty; make reasonable suspicion determination as appropriate; transport employee to collection site; notify Division Contact/DPC; prepare documentation.

— Determine if accident meets regulatory definition of an accident; if so transport employee to collection site or arrange for collections to be made; document test decision; notify Division Contact/DPC.

---

[7] City of Albuquerque
[8] City of Albuquerque

Figure B-11. Drug and Alcohol Testing Log[9]

<u>DRUG AND ALCOHOL TESTING LOG</u>

SS#	EE#	CLASS	AREA	DATE SCREENED	LOCATION	REASON
NAME:						
DRUG SCREEN/RESULTS	DATE	COMMENTS		ALCOHOL SCREEN RESULTS	DATE	COMMENTS

SS#	EE#	CLASS	AREA	DATE SCREENED	LOCATION	REASON
NAME:						
DRUG SCREEN/RESULTS	DATE	COMMENTS		ALCOHOL SCREEN RESULTS	DATE	COMMENTS

SS#	EE#	CLASS	AREA	DATE SCREENED	LOCATION	REASON
NAME:						
DRUG SCREEN/RESULTS	DATE	COMMENTS		ALCOHOL SCREEN RESULTS	DATE	COMMENTS

SS#	EE#	CLASS	AREA	DATE SCREENED	LOCATION	REASON
NAME:						
DRUG SCREEN/RESULTS	DATE	COMMENTS		ALCOHOL SCREEN RESULTS	DATE	COMMENTS

SS#	EE#	CLASS	AREA	DATE SCREENED	LOCATION	REASON
NAME:						
DRUG SCREEN/RESULTS	DATE	COMMENTS		ALCOHOL SCREEN RESULTS	DATE	COMMENTS

SS#	EE#	CLASS	AREA	DATE SCREENED	LOCATION	REASON
NAME:						
DRUG SCREEN/RESULTS	DATE	COMMENTS		ALCOHOL SCREEN RESULTS	DATE	COMMENTS

---

[9] Massachusetts Bay Transportation Authority (MBTA)

Figure B-12. Drug Test Result Summary Form[10]

DRUG TEST RESULT SUMMARY FORM

To Be Completed By MRO

Company: _____

Location: _____

Employee Name: _____

Identification #: _____

Reported for Test: _____ Date _____ Time

Specimen Collection: _____ Date _____ Time

Type of Test:
- _____ Pre-Employment _____ Return-to-Duty
- _____ Random _____ Post-Accident
- _____ Reasonable Suspicion _____ Follow-up
- _____ Re-Test _____ Other

Type of Test: _____ DOT _____ Safe 10 _____ Safe 5 _____ Other

Date Lab Received: _____

Date Lab Reported: _____

Date MRO Verifies Results: _____

Specimen Collection Site:
- Name: _____
- Location: _____
- Technician: _____

Testing Laboratory:
- Name: _____
- Location: _____
- Certifying Scientist: _____

Split Analysis Laboratory:
- Name: _____
- Location: _____
- Certifying Scientist: _____

Medical Review Officer:
- Name: _____
- Location: _____
- Signature: _____

Test Result:
- _____ Negative _____ Positive _____ Unsuitable _____ Not Performed
- _____ Cancelled _____ Insufficient Volume _____ Adulterated

Substance Detected:
- _____ Marijuana _____ Cocaine _____ Phencyclidine
- _____ Opiates _____ Amphetamine _____ Other, Specify:
- _____ Codeine _____ Amphetamine
- _____ Morphine _____ Methamphetamine

Date Employee Informed: _____

Action Taken:
- _____ Referred to SAP (Date) _____ _____ Employee Terminated
- _____ Assigned to non-safety-sensitive duties _____ Not Hired
- _____ Removed from Duty _____ Other

---

[10] City of Albuquerque

Figure B-13. Supervisor Log for Drug and Alcohol Testing[11] (Front)

SUPERVISOR LOG – DRUG & ALCOHOL TESTING

DATE _____ EMPLOYEE NAME _____

SSN / ID# OF EMPLOYEE _____

EMPLOYEE WORK SITE_____

TYPE OF TEST

☐ DRUG ☐ ALCOHOL ☐ BOTH DRUG & ALCOHOL

REASON FOR TESTING

☐ RANDOM ☐ REASONABLE SUSPICION

☐ POST-ACCIDENT ☐ FOLLOW-UP (per return-to-work agreement)

TESTING FACILITY

☐ MEDWORK (SR-84) ☐ ON-SITE (employee's work location)

☐ FAMILY HEALTH CENTER ☐ OTHER_____

(am/pm) ### SEQUENCE OF EVENTS

_____ Time when testing facility was called/notified to coordinate testing of a Mass Transit Division employee.
_____ Time when employee was first notified of the testing requirement.
_____ Time when union/other employee representative was contacted (person notified) _____).
_____ Departure time from employee's work site to the testing facility, if applicable.
_____ Arrival time at the testing facility, or time the mobile testing team arrives at the testing location.
_____ Arrival time of union representative, if applicable.
_____ Time testing started.
_____ Time testing concluded.
_____ Time of return to work location, or time employee is released to return to duty or is secured from duty.

OTHER NOTIFICATION
(post-accident, reasonable suspicion testing, or as otherwise required)

_____ Time when Superintendent/Assistant Superintendent was notified.
_____ Time when Program Manager for Drug & Alcohol Testing was called/alerted.
_____ Time when Director/Assistant Director was notified, if applicable.
_____ Other _____

[11] Broward County (Florida) Transit

Figure B-13. Supervisor Log for Drug and Alcohol Testing (Back)

POST-ACCIDENT TESTING

(Complete this section only if post-accident testing criteria applies.)

_____   _____   ☐   BODILY INJURY
(Date/Time of Accident)   *(Location of Accident)*

☐   DISABLING DAMAGE

☐   **NO-TEST DECISION** (WAIVED PER _____)

_____

REASONABLE SUSPICION TESTING

(Complete this section to describe when, where, and what specific, <u>observed</u> behavior, speech, appearance, or other characteristic results in a reasonable suspicion testing determination. <u>Be specific.</u> Use amplifying comments or separate sheet of paper if more space is needed.)

_____   _____   ☐   ODOR OF ALCOHOL
(Date/Time of Observation)   *(Location of Observation)*

_____

_____

AMPLIFYING COMMENTS

(Complete this section to note any problem or unusual circumstance associated with the testing process, any delay in testing beyond two hours of notifying employee of a testing requirement, or to provide additional information, if needed. Use continuation sheet if more space is needed.)

_____

_____

_____

_____

_____

_____

_____

_____
(Signature of Supervisor)

<u>Note</u>. *Post-Accident and Reasonable Suspicion testing must be substantiated by completing the appropriate section above. Return this form within 24 hours of testing to the Program Manager for Drug and Alcohol Testing, Broward County Transit, 3201 West Copans Road, Pompano Beach, Florida 33069. Contact the Program Manager at 357-830., After regular business hours call 497-8327 (24-hour pager) if there is question concerning this form or assistance is needed in determining whether a particular situation requires testing for the use of prohibited drugs or misuse of alcohol.*

Figure B-14. Order for Testing[12]

ORDER FOR TESTING

Name: _____

Number: _____

Supervisor Authorizing Test: _____

Collection Site: _____

_____

Transported: ____ Yes ____ No

Name of Transport
Supervisor: _____

Date & Time Sent: _____ (Date) _____ (Time)

Test Authority: ___ DOT   ____ Non-DOT   ____ Other (Specify)

Test Category:
     ___ Pre-employment   ____ Random
     ___ Post-Accident   ____ Reasonable Suspicion
     ___ Return-to-Duty   ____ Follow-up
     ___ Retest

Observed Collection: ___ Yes   ____ No

Other _____

_____

Special
Instructions: _____

Date & Time Sent: _____ Date   _____ Time
Date & Time Reported: _____ Date   _____ Time
Date & Time of Test: _____ Date   _____ Time

---

[12] Ohio Department of Transportation (ODOT)

Figure B-15. Notification of Testing

**MV TRANSPORTATION
DRUG & ALCOHOL TESTING
NOTIFICATION FORM**

Employee Identification
Employee Name:
Employee ID No: (ss#)
Department:
Supervisor:

TYPE OF TEST	DRUG _____ ALCOHOL _____
RANDOM	
POST ACCIDENT	DOT NON-DOT
REASONABLE SUSPICION	
RETURN TO STUDY	
FOLLOW UP	

Selection, Notification, and Testing	
For MVT Use	This side to be filled out by collection site staff
Date Selected:	Date Tested:
Date Notified:	Time Tested: am/pm
Time Notified: am/pm	Location:

_____   _____
Employer Signature   **Date**

_____   _____
Collection Person Signature   **Date**

Figure B-16. Notice of Positive Drug Test[13]

HUMAN RESOURCES - DEPARTMENT #6210
NOTICE OF POSITIVE DRUG TES

CONFIDENTIAL

DATE: June 5, 2002

TO: ____, Manager, _____

FROM: _____ Drug and Alcohol Program Coordinator

SUBJ: ____, Badge #___

____, Badge #___, had a drug test on ____, 2001 at ____ Medical Clinic. The test results for both were verified positive for Marijuana (THC) on ____, 2001. A copy of the Medical Review Officer's (MRO) Status Report is attached.

To assist you with preparing for disciplinary action, the following checklist of mandatory actions is included:

☐ Remove the employee from duty.   Date of removal from duty: _____

☐ Notify the employee of the test result.

☐ Refer employee to Employee Assistance Program (EAP) for assessment by a Substance Abuse Professional (SAP) and treatment resource information (Initial referral), this must be done regardless of disciplinary action to be taken, in order to be in compliance with DOT/FTA regulations and the MTA/PTSC Alcohol-and Drug-Free Work Environment Policy.)

☐ Schedule a disciplinary hearing.   Date of hearing: _____

☐ Ask if employee requested the Split Sample test. *(As this test can only be performed at the employee's written request, this serves only as a reminder.)* **Have employee sign the Authorization to Release Drug Test Result to Union**, (required by some unions in order to pay for the Split Sample test.)

☐ Contact _____ to schedule a meeting with the Discipline Committee, as soon as the hearing date is set.

A copy of this completed form and of the final disciplinary action taken <u>must be sent to this office</u>, as soon as a decision has been made and all parties notified.

Thanks for your cooperation. If you have any questions regarding this matter, please call me at _____.

Attachments

---

[13] Los Angeles County Metropolitan Transportation Authority (LACMTA)

Figure B-17. Notice of Positive Alcohol Test[14]

HUMAN RESOURCES - DEPARTMENT #6210
NOTICE OF POSITIVE ALCOHOL TEST

CONFIDENTIAL

DATE: June 5, 2002

TO: ____, Manager, Division ____

FROM: ____, Drug and Alcohol Program Coordinator

SUBJ: ____, Badge #___

____, Badge #___ had a Breathalyzer test ___day, ____, 2001, at _____ Industrial Medical Clinic. The initial test result had an alcohol concentration of **0. 0**___ and was confirmed positive by a second test at **0.0**__. A copy of the test results is attached. We are still awaiting drug test results and they will be reported to you, as soon as they are available.

To assist you with preparing for disciplinary action, the following checklist of mandatory actions is included:

☐ Remove the employee from duty.   Date of removal from duty _____

☐ Notify the employee of the test result.

☐ Refer employee to Employee Assistance Program (EAP) for assessment by a Substance Abuse Professional (SAP) and treatment resource information (Initial referral), this <u>must</u> be done regardless of disciplinary action to be taken, to be in compliance with the MTA/PTSC Alcohol-and Drug-Free Work Environment Policy.)

☐ Schedule a disciplinary hearing. Date of hearing: _____

☐ Contact ____ to schedule a meeting with the Discipline Committee, as soon as the hearing date is set.

A copy of this completed form and of the final disciplinary action taken <u>must be sent to this office</u>, as soon as a decision has been made and all parties notified.

Thanks for your cooperation. If you have any question regarding this matter, please call me at ____.

Attachments

---

[14] Los Angeles County Metropolitan Transportation Authority (LACMTA)

Figure B-18. Employee Notification of Positive Test Result[15]

Employee Notification of a Positive Drug/Alcohol Screen

Employee Name: _____

Employee Identification Number: _____

Attached is a copy of your positive drug and/or alcohol screen. This information (not the actual test result) is being forwarded to your supervisor for appropriate action.

YOU MUST REPORT TO YOUR SUPERVISOR _____, **AT**

$\qquad\qquad\qquad\qquad\qquad\qquad$ **(Supervisor's Name)**

_____**IMMEDIATELY UPON RELEASE**

(Location employee must report to.)

FROM THE CLINIC.

If you fail to report to the supervisor, additional disciplinary action may be imposed, up to and including discharge.

Notice of Availability of Substance Abuse Professional Evaluation

A Substance Abuse Professional evaluation is available for you. Please contact the MBTA Employee Assistance Program (EAP) to schedule an appointment. (617) 222-5381. The MBTA EAP is located at 120 Boylston Street, 6th Floor, Boston, MA. (across the hall from the MBTA clinic.) In the case of an emergency, contact the 24-hour pager (781) 553-0001.

_____   _____   _____
Employee Signature   **Date**   **Time**

_____   _____
Print Employee Name   **Witness**

---

[15]Massachusetts Bay Transportation Authority (MBTA)

Figure B-19. Supervisor Notification of Positive Test Result[16]

DRUG AND/OR ALCOHOL SCREEN INFORMATION FORM
SUPERVISOR NOTIFICATION

The following information is considered strictly **confidential.** It is being forwarded to you to ensure the employee is removed from safety-sensitive duties and to initiate the appropriate disciplinary action. **Each supervisor is responsible for ensuring that this information is filed in a confidential and secure area.** It may be released to additional management personnel on a need to know basis only.

EMPLOYEE IDENTIFICATION NUMBER: _____

DATE OF DRUG AND/OR ALCOHOL SCREEN: _____
    (INDICATE DRUG OR ALCOHOL)

REASON FOR DRUG/ALCOHOL SCREEN: _____
(FTA REQUIRED TEST ONLY)

MRO VERIFICATION DATE: _____

_____   _____
Authorized Medical Clinic Signature   **Date**

Pursuant to the MBTA Drug and Alcohol Policy and Testing Program, effective August 1, 2001. An employee must be instructed to comply with Section V, Enforcement of Policy Through Discipline. This section includes, but is not limited to, the supervisor instructing the employee that he or she **must report** to the MBTA Employee Assistance Program for a Substance Abuse Professional Evaluation as required by 49 CFR part 40.

As a supervisor you **may** contact the MBTA Employee Assistance Program to schedule an evaluation or you **must** instruct the employee that he/she must complete the evaluation within seven (7) days of the discipline being issued.

Please contact the MBTA Employee Assistance Program, 120 Boylston Street, 6th Floor, Boston, MA. (617) 222-5381, to schedule a Substance Abuse Professional Evaluation.

_____   _____
Employee Signature   Date

_____
Witness

_____
[16]Massachusetts Bay Transportation Authority (MBTA)

PRE-EMPLOYMENT TESTING

Figure B-20. Flow Chart for Pre-Employment Testing Process[17]

FTA DRUG & ALCOHOL TESTING PROGRAM

Pre-Employment Testing

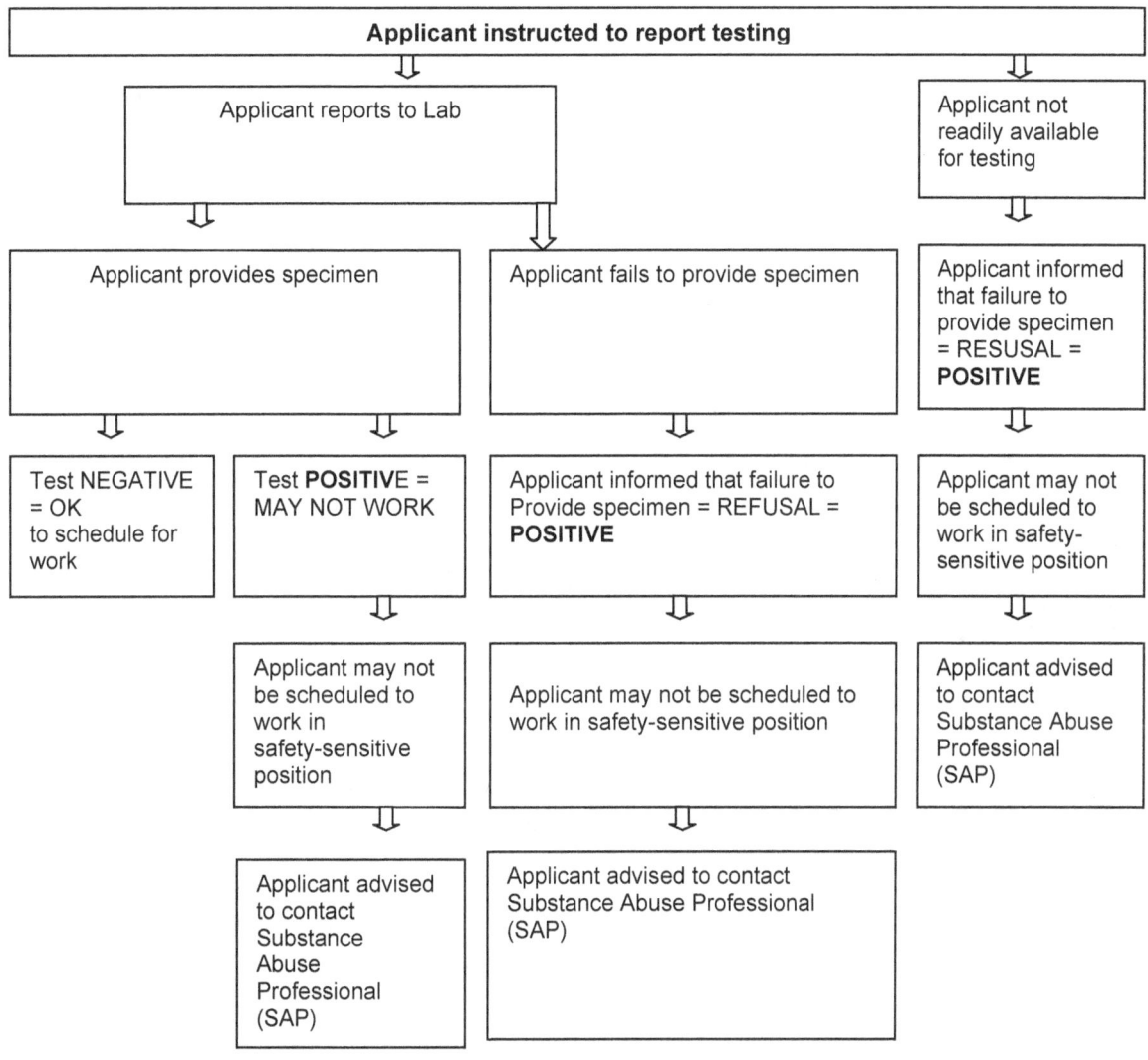

Figure B-21. Pre-Employment Documentation Summary Sheet[18]

PRE-EMPLOYMENT DOCUMENTATION
SUMMARY SHEET

Applicant Name: _____

Address: _____

City/State/Zip: _____
_____

Telephone: _____

Date of Application: _____

Position Applied For:

_____ CDL, Specify _____

_____ Public Safety

       _____ Police

       _____ Fire

       _____ Correction

       _____ Other, Specify _____

_____ Transit

       _____ Operator

       _____ Dispatcher

       _____ Mechanic

       _____ Security w/ Firearm

       _____ Other, Specify _____

_____ Other, Specify _____

For Transit Only:
Safety-Sensitive Job Function:

       _____ Operate a revenue service vehicle

       _____ CDL for non-revenue service vehicle

       _____ Maintenance of revenue service vehicle

       _____ Controlling movement of revenue service vehicle

       _____ Security with firearm

Date of Applicant Notification: _____

Date of Test: _____

Date Reported to Department: _____

Date of Hire: _____

Test Result: Positive _____   Negative _____   Canceled _____

Attachments: ☐ Notification (F-3)   ☐ Chain of Custody (COC7)

                  ☐ Test Result Summary Form (F-4)   ☐ Order to Test (F-22)

---

[18] City of Albuquerque

Figure B-22. Pre-Employment Test Tracking Log [19]

PRE –EMPLOYMENT TEST TRACKING LOG

Name of Applicant	Notification of Test	Date of Test	Consent Form	COC Form	Test Result	Date Result Reported	Hire Date	Comment

---

[19] City of Albuquerque

Figure B-23. Applicant Notification of Positive Test Result[20]

Applicant Notification of a Positive Drug/Alcohol Screen

Applicant Name: _____

Applicant Identification Number: _____
  (Social Security #)

Attached is a copy of your positive drug and/or alcohol screen. This information (not the actual test result) is being forwarded to the Human Resources Department for appropriate action.

Human Resources Representative _____

Telephone # _____

Notice of Availability of Substance Abuse Professional Evaluation

A Substance Abuse Professional evaluation is available for you. Please contact the MBTA Employee Assistance Program (EAP) to schedule an appointment. (617) 222-5381. The MBTA EAP is located at 120 Boylston Street, 6th Floor, Boston, MA. (across the hall from the MBTA clinic.) In the case of an emergency contact the 24-hour pager (781) 553-0001.

_____   _____   _____
Applicant Signature   Date   Time

_____   _____
Print Applicant Name   Witness

---

[20]Massachusetts Bay Transportation Authority (MBTA)

REASONABLE SUSPICION TESTING

Figure B-24. Flow Chart for Reasonable Suspicion Testing Process[21]

FTA DRUG & ALCOHOL TESTING PROGRAM

Reasonable Suspicion Testing

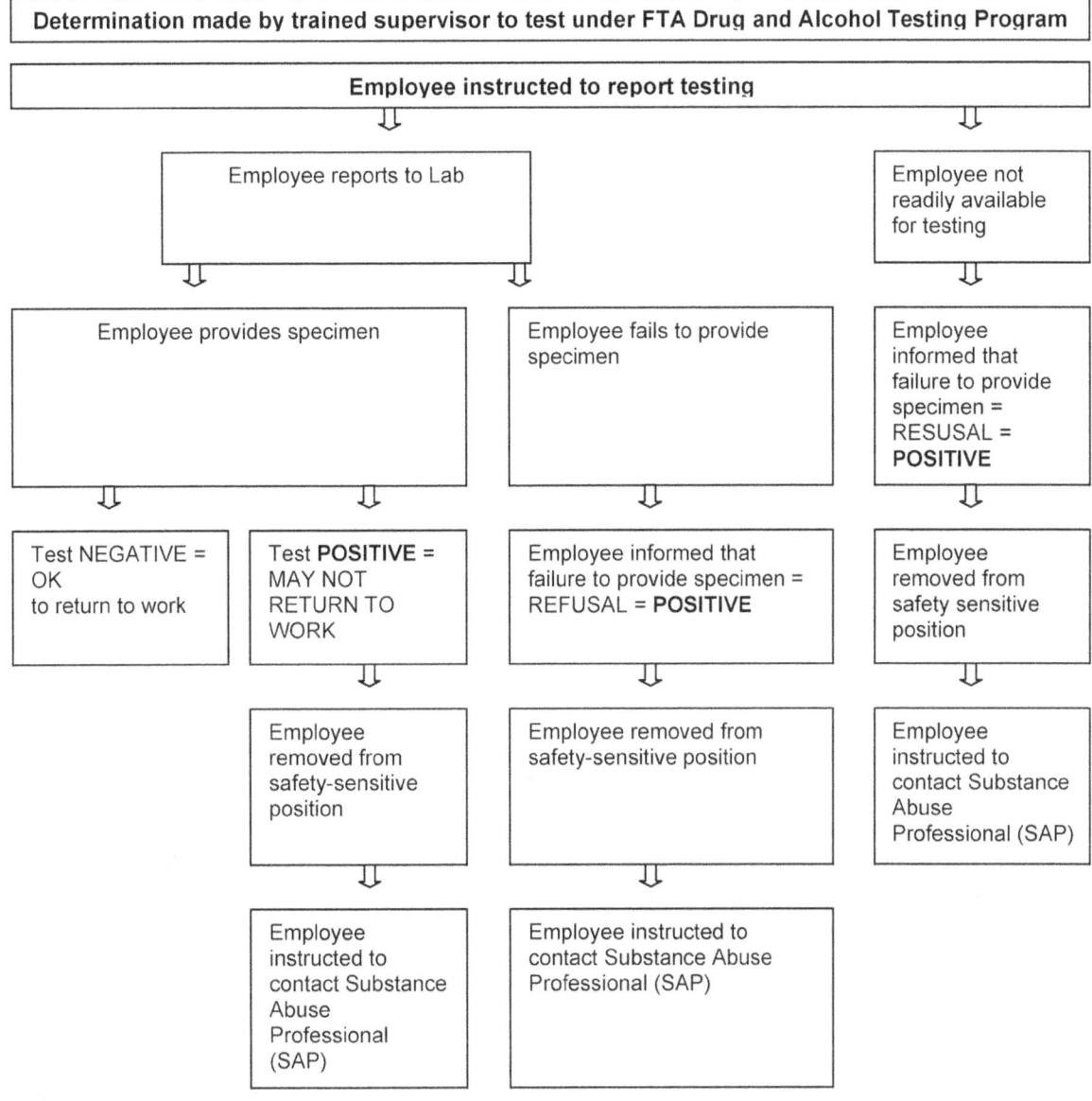

---

[21] West Virginia Department of Transportation (DOT), Division of Public Transit

Figure B-25. Reasonable Suspicion Process and Documentation[22] (Sheet 1)

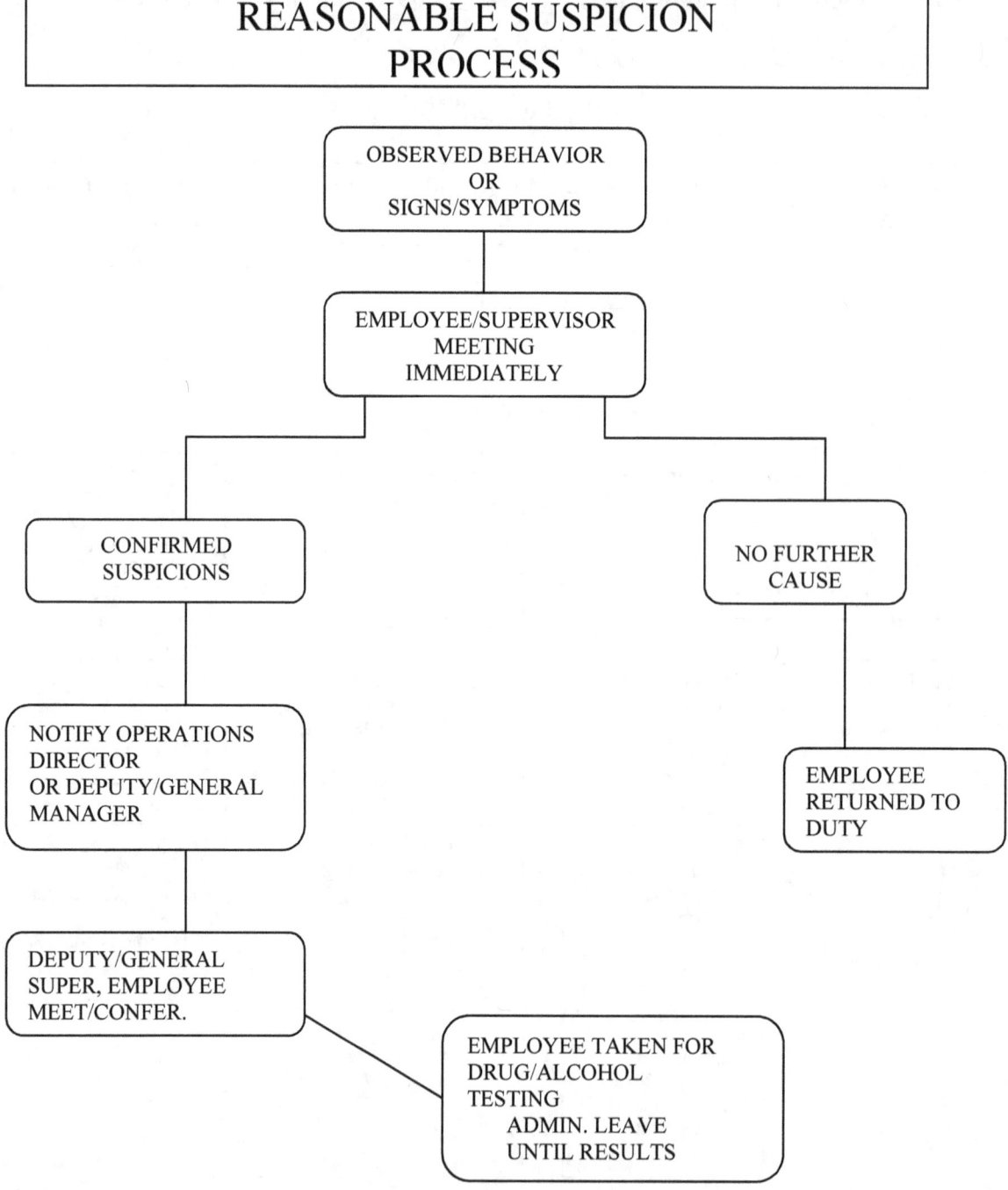

REASONABLE SUSPICION
PROCESS

OBSERVED BEHAVIOR
OR
SIGNS/SYMPTOMS

EMPLOYEE/SUPERVISOR
MEETING
IMMEDIATELY

CONFIRMED
SUSPICIONS

NO FURTHER
CAUSE

NOTIFY OPERATIONS
DIRECTOR
OR DEPUTY/GENERAL
MANAGER

EMPLOYEE
RETURNED TO
DUTY

DEPUTY/GENERAL
SUPER, EMPLOYEE
MEET/CONFER.

EMPLOYEE TAKEN FOR
DRUG/ALCOHOL
TESTING
    ADMIN. LEAVE
    UNTIL RESULTS

---

[22] Western Maine Transportation Services

Figure B-25. Reasonable Suspicion Process and Documentation (Sheet 2)

Western Maine Transportation Services
REASONABLE SUSPICION DOCUMENTATION FORM

EMPLOYEE NAME	DATE OF OBSERVATION (MONTH, DAY, YEAR)
LOCATION	TIME OF OBSERVATION FROM AM PM TO AM PM

OBSERVED PERSONAL BEHAVIOR (CHECK ALL APPROPRIATE ITEMS)

BREATH: (Odor of alcoholic beverage)	☐ STRONG ☐ NONE	☐ FAINT	☐ MODERATE
EYES:	☐ BLOODSHOT ☐ CLEAR ☐ DILATED PUPILS	☐ GLASSY ☐ HEAVY EYELIDS	☐ NORMAL ☐ FIXED PUPILS
SPEECH:	☐ CONFUSED ☐ ACCENT ☐ SLURRED ☐ NOT UNDERSTANDABLE	☐ STUTTERED ☐ MUMBLED ☐ GOOD ☐ COTTON MOUTHED	☐ THICK TONGUED ☐ FAIR ☐ MUSH MOUTHED ☐ OTHER:
ATTITUDE:	☐ EXCITED ☐ INDIFFFERENT ☐ CARE FREE ☐ COOPERATIVE OTHER:	☐ COMBATIVE ☐ TALKATIVE ☐ COCKY ☐ PROFANE	☐ HILARIOUS ☐ INSULTING ☐ SLEEPY ☐ POLITE
UNUSUAL ACTION:	☐ HICCOUGHING ☐ FIGHTING ☐ OTHER:	☐ BELCHING ☐ CRYING	☐ VOMITING ☐ LAUGHING
BALANCE:	☐ FALLING ☐ SWAYING	☐ NEEDS SUPPORT ☐ OTHER:	☐ WOBBLING
WALKING:	☐ FALLING ☐ SWAYING	☐ STAGGERING ☐ OTHER	☐ STUMBLING
TURNING	☐ FALLING ☐ SWAYING	☐ STAGGERING ☐ HESITANT	☐ STUMBLING ☐ OTHER:
ANY OTHER UNUSUAL ACTIONS OR STATEMENTS:			

SIGNS OR COMPLAINTS OF ILLNESS OR INJURY:

SUPERVISOR'S OPINION

EFFECTS OF ALCOHOL/DRUG INTOXICATION	☐ NONE ☐ EXTREME	☐ SLIGHT	☐ OBVIOUS
OPERATION OF EQUIPMENT	☐ YES ☐ NO	COMMENTS:	
ADDITIONAL COMMENTS:			

SUPERVISOR	SIGNATURE	DATE	TIME
WITNESS	WITNESS	WITNESS	

Figure B-26. Reasonable Suspicion Short-Term Indicators

LOS ANGELES COUNTY METROPOLITAN TRANSPORTATION AUTHORITY

REASONABLE SUSPICION SHORT-TERM INDICATORS

Manager/Supervisor: This form is to be used to substantiate and document the objective facts and circumstances leading to a reasonable suspicion determination. After careful observation of the employee's behavior, please check **all** of the short-term indicators that denote a possible link to the employee's use of prohibited alcohol or drugs.

Employee Name_____ Badge _____ Job Title _____Dept._____

Supervisor Name_____ Badge _____ Telephone _____

Second Supervisor_____(if applicable) Badge_____

A. Incident/Cause for Suspicion
- ☐ Apparent drug or alcohol intoxication
- ☐ Abnormal or erratic behavior
- ☐ Observed/reported possession, dispensation or use of a prohibited substance
- ☐ Arrest or conviction for drug-related offense(s)

B. Body Behavior
- ☐ Nausea or vomiting
- ☐ Extreme fatigue/sleeping on job
- ☐ Dizziness or fainting
- ☐ Highly excited or nervous
- ☐ Odor of alcohol

C. Body Appearance
- ☐ Either very flushed or very pale
- ☐ Excessive sweating or skin clamminess
- ☐ Dry mouth, frequent swallowing, wetting lips frequently
- ☐ Disheveled appearance/out of uniform

D. Body Movements
- ☐ Unsteady walk, poor coordination
- ☐ Shaking hands/body, tremors, twitches
- ☐ Breathing irregularly, or with difficulty
- ☐ Loss of physical control

E. Eyes
- ☐ Bloodshot or watery
- ☐ Dilated or constricted pupils

F. Speech
- ☐ Slurred or incoherent speech
- ☐ Repetitious, rambles

G. Behavioral Indicators Noted
- ☐ Verbal abusiveness
- ☐ Physical abusiveness
- ☐ Extreme aggressiveness or unresponsiveness
- ☐ Inappropriate response to questioning or instructions
- ☐ Erratic/inappropriate behavior, hallucinations, disorientation, confusion, talkativeness, euphoric - (Circle all that apply)

Written summary including any pertinent information not noted above_____
_____
_____
_____

Reasonable Suspicion Test Performed **Yes**☐ **No**☐ Date ___/___/___ Time _____

Clinic_____

Reasonable Suspicion Test Refused **Yes**☐ **No**☐ Date ___/___/___ Time _____

Signature of Supervisor _____ Date ___/___/___ Time _____

Figure B-27. Reasonable Suspicion Evaluation and Checklist[23] (Sheet 1)

This form is required to be completed by the supervisor of a safety-sensitive employee as a guideline for the determination to order a drug and/or alcohol test screen for the employee when reasonable suspicion exists subject to the MBTA's Drug and Alcohol Policy. The supervisor or a responsible company official shall independently complete this form in its entirety.

Name of safety-sensitive employee: _____.

Employee identification number: _____

Position description of employee: _____

Date and time of evaluation: _____

Location of employee when reasonable suspicion evaluation was made: _____
_____(be specific)

Evaluating supervisor: _____

Other supervisors at the location: _____
_____

I.   CIRCUMSTANCES OCCURRING AT THE TIME OF THE EVALUATION

- ❏ Employee is reporting for duty: Yes   No   (circle one)
- ❏ Employee is already on duty: Yes   No   (circle one)

II.   OBSERVATIONS OF EMPLOYEE'S PHYSICAL CONDITION

Check below any/all applicable behaviors and describe:

____ Slurred speech   _____

____ Confusion / disorientation   _____

____ Odor of alcohol on breath or person   _____

____ Odor of marijuana on breath or person   _____

____ Unsteady gait or lack of balance   _____

____ Glassy eyes   _____

____ Rapid or continuous eye movement or inability
to focus   _____

____ Drowsiness   _____

---

[23]Massachusetts Bay Transportation Authority (MBTA)

Figure B-27. Reasonable Suspicion Evaluation and Checklist (Sheet 2)

____ Inattentiveness   _____

____ Apparent intoxicated behavior (without the odor of alcohol or marijuana   _____

____ Apparent intoxicated behavior (without the odor of alcohol or marijuana)   _____

____ Physical injury. Indicate location on body: _____

____ Tremors or bodily shaking   _____

____ Poor concentration   _____

____ Runny nose or sores around nostrils   _____

____ Very large or very small eye pupils   _____

____ Slow or inappropriate reactions   _____

III.   OBSERVATIONS OF EMPLOYEE'S BEHAVIOR

Check below any/all applicable behaviors and describe:

____ Inability to respond to questions or to respond correctly   _____

____ Complaints of racing or irregular heart beating   _____

____ Marked irritability   _____

____ Aggressiveness (attempts at physical contact)   _____

____ Inappropriate laughter, crying, etc.   _____

____ Sleeping on the job   _____

____ Fainting or repeated loss of consciousness   _____

____ Inappropriate job performance and/or violation of Authority rule(s)   _____

Figure B-27. Reasonable Suspicion Evaluation and Checklist (Sheet 3)

IV. DETERMINATION OF REASONABLE SUSPICION

Based on the above documented information, I have determined that there   is   is not   (supervisor to circle only one) reasonable suspicion for sending _____ for a FTA drug and alcohol screening test.

The drug and alcohol screening tests have been ordered by:_____.

To be conducted at: _____MBTA Medical Services
_____ Charlestown Garage
_____ Cabot Garage

Signature of supervisor/official conducting the evaluation: _____

Printed name of the supervisor conducting the evaluation and employee identification number:

_____

Date: _____ (month, day, year).

Figure B-28. Fitness for Duty[24] (Sheet 1)

FITNESS FOR DUTY

CONFIDENTIAL

EMPLOYEE   DATE/TIME OF INCIDENT

SUPERVISOR NAME AND TELEPHONE

This checklist is to be completed when an observation has occurred which provides reasonable suspicion that an employee is under the influence of a prohibited drug substance or alcohol. You should note all pertinent behavior and physical signs or symptoms, which lead you to reasonably believe that the employee has recently used or is under the influence of a prohibited substance. Mark each applicable item on this form and any additional facts or circumstances which you have noted.

A.   Nature of Incident/Cause for Suspicion

_____**1.**   Observed/reported possession or use of a prohibited substance (including passenger complaint)
_____**2.**   Apparent drug or alcohol intoxication
_____**3.**   Observed abnormal or erratic behavior
_____**4.**   Arrest or conviction for drug-related offense
_____**5.**   Other (e.g., flagrant violation of safety or serious misconduct, accident, or "near miss", fighting or argumentative/abusive language, refusal or supervisor instruction, unauthorized absence on the job). Please specify.

_____
_____
_____
_____
_____

B.   Behavioral Indicators Noted

_____**1.**   Verbal abusiveness
_____**2.**   Physical abusiveness
_____**3.**   Extreme aggressiveness or agitation
_____**4.**   Withdrawal, depression, tearfulness, or responsiveness
_____**5.**   Inappropriate verbal responses to questioning or instructions
_____**6.**   Paranoid
_____**7.**   Lethargic
_____**8.**   Other erratic or inappropriate behavior (e.g., hallucinations, disorientation, excessive euphoria, talkativeness, confusion). Please explain.

_____
_____
_____
_____
_____

---

[24] City of Albuquerque and Ohio Department of Transportation

Figure B-28. Fitness for Duty (Sheet 2)

C.   Physical Signs or Symptoms

_____	1.	Possession, dispensing, or using prohibited substance
_____	2.	Slurred or slowed speech
_____	3.	Incoherent, confused speech
_____	4.	Silent or whispering
_____	5.	Swaying, falling, staggering
_____	6.	Stumbling, reaching for support
_____	7.	Arm raised for balance
_____	8.	Unsteady gait or other loss of physical control, poor coordination
_____	9.	Dilated or constricted pupils or unusual eye movement
_____	10.	Bloodshot or watery eyes
_____	11.	Extreme aggressiveness or agitation
_____	12.	Excessive sweating or clamminess of skin
_____	13.	Flushed or very pale face
_____	14.	Highly excited or nervous
_____	15.	Nausea or vomiting
_____	16.	Odor of alcohol
_____	17.	Odor of marijuana
_____	18.	Disheveled appearance or out of uniform
_____	19.	Dry mouth (frequent swallowing/lip wetting)
_____	20.	Dizziness or fainting
_____	21.	Shaking hands or body tremors/twitching
_____	22.	Breathing irregularity or difficulty breathing
_____	23.	Runny nose or sores around nostrils
_____	24.	Inappropriate wearing of sunglasses
_____	25.	Puncture marks or "tracks"
_____	26.	Other (please specify)

_____
_____
_____

D.   Observation Summary

Speech: _____

Coordination: _____

Standing: _____

Walking/Turning: _____

Hand Movement: _____

Balance: _____

Figure B-28. Fitness for Duty (Sheet 3)

D.   Observation Summary (Continued)

Disorientation: _____

_____

Judgment/Decision Making: _____

_____

Appearance: _____

_____

Nose: _____

_____

Eyes: _____

_____

Skin: _____

_____

Clothing: _____

_____

Odor: _____

_____

Other: _____

_____

_____

E.   Written Summary

Please summarize the facts and circumstances of the incident, employee response, supervisor actions taken, and any other pertinent information not previously noted. Please note the date, times, and locations of reasonable suspicion testing or note if the employee refused the test. Attach additional sheets as needed.

_____

_____

_____

_____

_____

_____

_____

_____

_____

_____

_____   _____
Signature of Supervisor   **Date/Time**

_____   _____
Signature of Witness (if possible)   **Date/Time**

Figure B-29. Observation/Incident Report[25] (Front)

SUBSTANCE ABUSE PROGRAM
OBSERVATION / INCIDENT REPORT

☐ REASONABLE CAUSE ☐ POST-ACCIDENT ☐ RANDOM *(Check One)*

Date of Report_____ Date and Time of Incident_____

Location of Observation _____

Observing Supervisor _____

Name of Observed Employee_____

Reasonable Cause Testing

Reasonable cause for testing means suspicion based on specific personal observation by a supervisor or other company official trained in detecting the signs and symptoms of drug or alcohol abuse. The observer shall determine whether the employee is being tested under DOT/FTA mandate or District Policy and shall describe and document his/her findings.

DOT FTA Safety-Sensitive Employee Policy:
☐ Specific persons and articulable observations concerning the appearance, behavior, speech, or body odors of the employee.

District Policy All Employees:
☐ Violation of a safety rule, other unsafe work incident that leads supervisor to believe that drug/alcohol use may be a factor.

☐ Other physical, circumstantial or contemporaneous indicators of drug or alcohol use.

Post-Accident Testing

Any employee must submit to drug and/or alcohol testing after an accident, whenever a supervisor determines he/she contributed to the accident or cannot be completely discounted as a contributing factor to the accident. *Supervisor must indicate whether test is being conducted under DOT/FTA mandate or District Policy as defined below:*

DOT FTA Safety-Sensitive Employee Policy:
☐ A person dies testing is mandatory

☐ A person must be taken to a medical treatment facility

☐ Mass Transit vehicle removed from service due to damage

District Policy All Employees:
☐ A fatality

☐ A medical injury

☐ District property damage of $5,000 or more

Associated with the above mentioned kinds of behavior are a variety of "warning signs" that usually appear on the job.

PLACE A CHECK MARK √ NEXT TO THE SYMPTOM(S) OBSERVED IN THE ABOVE NAMED EMPLOYEE

	SYMPTOMS				
☐	Euphoria	☐	Exaggerated Sense of Ability	☐	Constricted Pupils
☐	Relaxed Inhibitions	☐	Drowsiness	☐	Dilated Pupils
☐	Slow/Depressed Breathing	☐	Depressed/Mood Changes	☐	Wandering Aimlessly
☐	Observed Use of Drugs	☐	Observed Use of Alcohol	☐	Disoriented Behavior
☐	Drunken Behavior (with or without smell of alcohol)	☐	Staggering Walk	☐	Odor of Alcohol
		☐	Slurred Speech	☐	Odor of Marijuana
☐	Rapid Breathing	☐	Excessively Talkative	☐	Hand Tremors
☐	Violent Behavior	☐	Combative/Argumentative	☐	Excessive Irritability
☐	Watery, Glassy, Red Eyes	☐	Staring into Space	☐	Poor Hand/Eye Coordination
☐	Hallucinations	☐	Poor Time Perception	☐	Other

---

[25] San Francisco Bay Area Rapid Transit (BART) District

Figure B-29. Observation/Incident Report (Back)

IF EMPLOYEE WILL BE TESTED:

1. If the employee is represented, the on-scene supervisor advises him/her of the right to have a union representative present prior to testing. Call for a union representative and document that union representation was called by the supervisor.

2. Order the employee to submit to a drug and alcohol test and to sign the consent and release forms. Advise him/her that failure to submit to a drug or alcohol test or failure to cooperate with the procedure is considered to be gross insubordination for failure to follow a direct order and will be cause for discipline up to and including discharge from District employment.

3. **For Reasonable Cause Testing Only:** Inform the employee of the availability of rehabilitation at the employee's own expense if the employee admits to drug or alcohol use prior to the test, if the employee is eligible, and inform the employee that a positive test will result in disciplinary action up to and including termination if the employee has not elected the rehabilitation option prior to the test.

4. Advise the employee that he/she will be in a paid status until the test sample is collected and the breath alcohol test is completed. The employee will then be placed in an unpaid status and relieved from duty until the District receives the drug test results. If both tests are negative, the District will make the employee whole.

DID EMPLOYEE ADMIT TO DRUG OR ALCOHOL USE:　　　　　　　YES　　　　NO

IF REASONABLE CAUSE, DID EMPLOYEE REQUEST REHABILITATION:　　YES　　　　NO

COMMENTS:_____
_____
_____
_____
_____

DESCRIBE INCIDENT: _____
_____
_____
_____
_____
_____
_____

ACTION TAKEN: _____
_____
_____
_____
_____

_____

SIGNATURE

ORIGINAL OF THIS REPORT TO MANAGER OF EMPLOYEE SERVICES
COPY OF THIS REPORT TO DEPARTMENT HEAD

Figure B-30. Accident/Incident/Reasonable Cause Report[26] (Front)

Accident/Incident/Reasonable Cause Report

PLEASE COMPLETE ALL AREAS NECESSARY ON THIS SIDE OF FORM

(X) areas that do not apply.

Employee:_____

Employee I.D. No._____

Division/Department:_____

Date of Accident/Incident:_____

Time:_____Location:_____

REVIEW THE REVERSE SIDE OF THIS FORM TO DETERMINE WHETHER THE TEST IS UNDER FTA OR RTD.

☐ **FTA-DOT** ☐ **RTD NON-DOT**

Remember, it is your responsibility to inform the person performing the test whether it is under FTA or RTD.

****

If you determine a test is not necessary, explain below:

A. Other than a fatality, if the accident falls within one of the categories on the reverse side, but you think the employee can be totally discounted you must complete the area below, explaining the accident and why you decided not to test.

_____

_____

_____

_____

****

B. Accidents or incidents where you believe negligence or carelessness may be involved. Briefly describe the accident/incident and why the employee may be under the influence of alcohol, drugs or a controlled substance. Complete the Reasonable Cause, Post Accident Section on the right side.

_____

_____

_____

_____

C. On-the-job accidents where serious injuries may have been caused by negligence or where more than one employee is involved, both the employee who caused the injury and the injured employee may be tested. Briefly descr be the accident and why you believe the employee may be under the influence of alcohol, drugs, or controlled substances. Complete the Reasonable Cause/Post Accident section on the right.

_____

_____

_____

_____

☐ **Reasonable Cause** ☐ **Post Accident**

Whether testing or not, this side must be completed. Complete each area on this side of the form.

Do Not Use N/A, O.K. or Leave Blank

If poss ble, a second supervisor should be retained as an additional witness.

_____
(Employee Name)

Speech:_____

_____

_____

Dexterity: (Standing/Walking)_____

_____

_____

Judgment/Decision Making:_____

_____

_____

Appearance: (eyes, clothing, etc.)_____

_____

_____

Odor: (alcoholic beverage, marijuana, etc.)____

_____

_____

Interpersonal interactions: (sudden outburst, mood swings, incoherent speech, etc.)

_____

_____

Other: (physical, verbal altercations, drug paraphernalia, etc.)

_____

_____

RTD Representative:_____

Date:_____

☐ **Sent for Testing** ☐ **Not Sent for Testing**

---

[26] Denver Regional Transit District

Figure B-30. Accident/Incident/Reasonable Cause Report (Back)

Under Federal regulations an incident is considered an accident if:

A. An individual dies.

B. An individual suffers bodily injury and is transported from the scene for immediate medical treatment.

C. The mass transit vehicle involved is a bus, electric bus, van, or automobile in which one or more vehicles incurs disabling damage as the result of the accident and must be transported from the scene by a tow truck or other vehicle.

D. The mass transit vehicle involved is a railcar, trolley car, trolley bus, or vessel, and is removed from revenue service.

*IF THE RTD EMPLOYEE INVOLVED IN THE ACCIDENT CAN BE TOTALLY DISCOUNTED AS A CONTRIBUTING FACTOR IN ITEMS B, C, AND D ONLY, THE EMPLOYEE DOES NOT HAVE TO BE TESTED. HOWEVER, FULL DOCUMENTATION MUST BE PROVIDED AS TO WHY THE TEST WAS NOT CONDUCTED.

Reasonable Suspicion Testing

The trained supervisors observe the employee and determines if testing is necessary based on specific, contemporaneously articulable observations concerning appearance, behavior, speech, or body odor of the employee.

ANYTIME TESTING IS NOT COMPLETED WITHIN TWO HOURS AFTER THE ACCIDENT OR INCIDENT YOU <u>MUST</u> DOCUMENT THE REASON.

Figure B-31. Reasonable Suspicion Individual Test Summary[27]

REASONABLE SUSPICION INDIVIDUAL TEST SUMMARY

TO BE COMPLETED BY SUPERVISOR

Employee Name: _____

Safety Sensitive Position: _____

Observation Date: _____ **Time:** _____

Circumstances of Observation: _____
(Attach additional sheets as necessary)

Objective Facts Identified (Attach additional sheets as necessary)

Behavior: _____

Appearance: _____

Speech: _____

Odor: _____

Other: _____

Safety-Sensitive Function Performed: _____

Notification Date: _____ **Time:** _____

Drug Test Date: _____ **Time:** _____

Alcohol Test Date: _____ **Time:** _____

Type of Test Conducted: _____ Drug _____ Alcohol

Supervisor Name: _____

Supervisor's Signature: _____

Did the alcohol test occur more than two hours from the time of the reasonable suspicion observation?

Yes _____ No _____ If yes, explain: _____

TO BE COMPLETED BY SUPERVISOR

If no alcohol test occurred because more than eight hours elapsed from the time of the reasonable suspicion observation, please explain: _____

If no drug test was performed because more than 32 hours had passed since the time of the reasonable suspicion observation, please explain: _____

Return the Form to your Department Program Coordinator within 24 hours.

TO BE COMPLETED BY THE SAPM

Date of Supervisor Training: _____

Test Results:				
Drug:	Positive _____	Negative _____	Canceled	
Alcohol:	Positive _____	Negative _____	0.02 - 0.039	

Comment: _____

Attachments: ☐ Test Result Summary Form   (F4)   ☐ Order to Test (F22)   ☐ Other
☐ Chain of Custody   ☐ Alcohol Test Form

---

[27] City of Albuquerque

Figure B-32. Reasonable Suspicion Tracking Master Log [28]

REASONABLE SUSPICION TRACKING MASTER LOG

Employee Name	Observation		Notification		Test		Notify SAPM (F-11)	Supervisor	Type Of Test [*]	Test Result (F-4) [**]	Alcohol Test Result (BATI) [**]
	Time	Date	Time	Date	Time	Date					

[*] Type Of Test: D - Drug; A - Alcohol

[**] Test Result: P - Positive; N - Negative; C - Cancelled

Figure B-33. Failure To Administer Reasonable Suspicion Drug Test Form[29]

PREPARE THIS FORM ONLY WHEN THE EMPLOYEE IS NOT TESTED WITHIN 32 HOURS OF THE DETERMINATION OF REASONABLE SUSPICION.

Name of safety-sensitive employee: _____
(first name, middle initial, last name)

Date of determination: _____ (month, day, year)

Time: _____ AM   PM   (circle one)

Location of employee when reasonable suspicion determination was made:

_____
_____
_____ (be specific)

Reason why the drug test was not administered (check all that apply):

❏ Safety-sensitive employee refused to be tested.
❏ Safety-sensitive employee was medically incapacitated.
❏ Safety-sensitive employee was arrested.
❏ Safety-sensitive employee was detained by law enforcement official.
❏ Other: _____

Specific disciplinary action (if any) taken by _____ (insert name of transit system, state, contractor or sub-recipient):

_____
_____
_____
_____

Date on which this report is completed: _____ (month, day, year).

Name of company official completing and filing report:
_____ (first name, middle initial, last name).

Title of company official completing and filing report:
_____

NOTE: _____ (INSERT NAME OF TRANSIT SYSTEM, STATE, CONTRACTOR, OR SUB-RECIPIENT) IS REQUIRED, WHEN THE ACCIDENT SATISFIES ONE OR MORE OF THE FTA THRESHOLDS, TO CONDUCT THE APPROPRIATE DRUG TEST. THE RESULTS OF A DRUG TEST CONDUCTED BY A LAW ENFORCEMENT OFFICIAL CAN BE SUBSTITUTED ONLY IF THE EMPLOYEE IS BEING DETAINED BY A LAW ENFORCEMENT OFFICIAL AND CAN NOT BE ACCESSED BY _____ (INSERT NAME OF TRANSIT SYSTEM, STATE, CONTRACTOR, OR SUB-RECIPIENT).

---

[29] SuTran Transit System, Sioux Falls, South Dakota

POST-ACCIDENT TESTING

Figure B-34. Post-Accident Test Decision Tree[30] (Front)

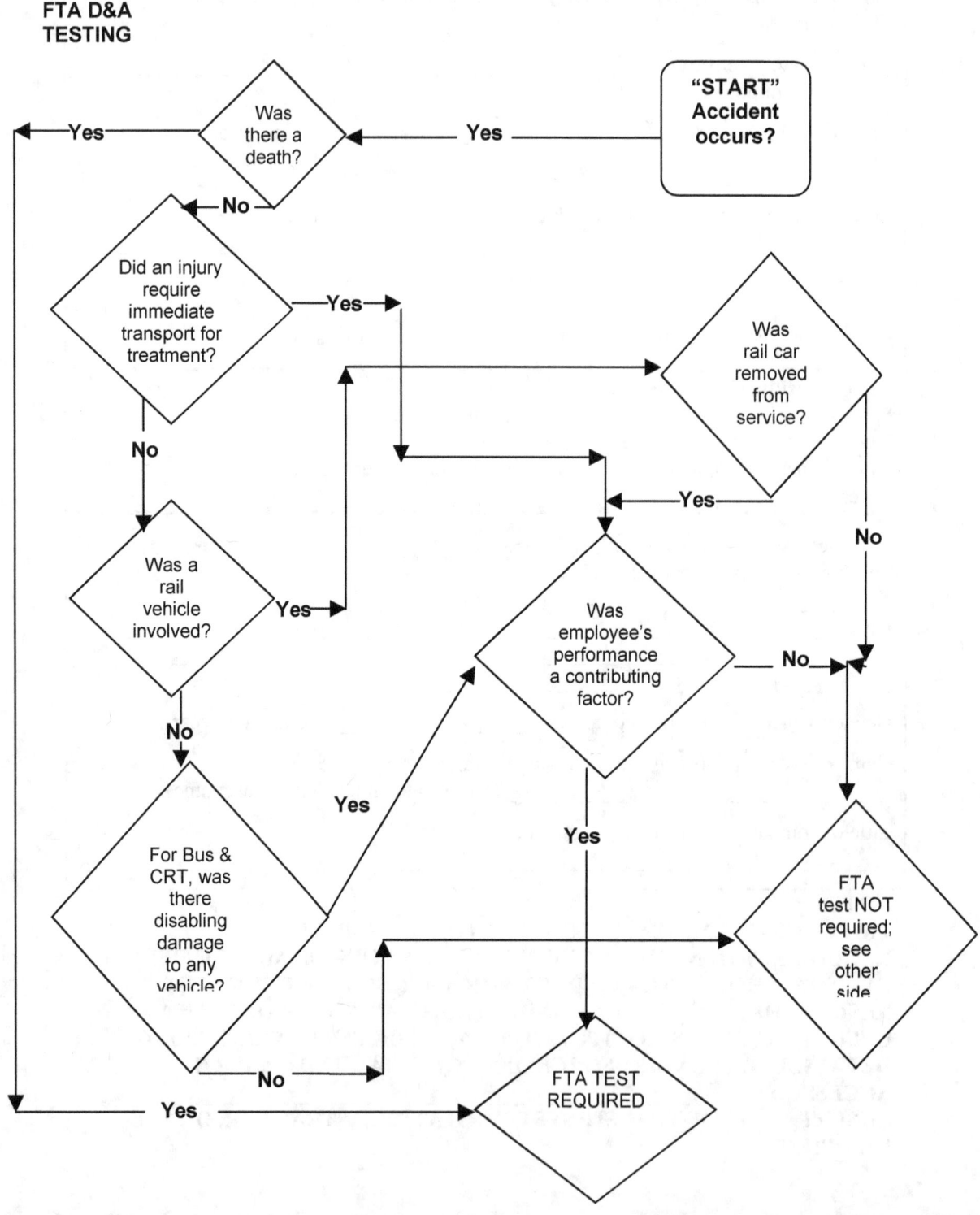

FTA D&A TESTING

"START" Accident occurs?

Yes → Was there a death?

Yes →

No ↓

Did an injury require immediate transport for treatment?

Yes →

No ↓

Was a rail vehicle involved?

Yes →

No ↓

For Bus & CRT, was there disabling damage to any vehicle?

Yes →

No →

Was rail car removed from service?

Yes →

No ↓

Was employee's performance a contributing factor?

No →

Yes ↓

FTA test NOT required; see other side

FTA TEST REQUIRED

Figure B-34. Post-Accident Test Decision Tree (Back)

RTA REQUIRED TESTING
(Safety Sensitive Only)

The following incidents require drug and alcohol testing by GCRTA policy when an employee either contributed to or cannot immediately be discounted from contributing to the accident, involving:

- **A pedestrian**

- **A fixed object**

- **Two or more GCRTA vehicles**

- **A GCRTA vehicle striking the rear end of another vehicle**

- **A head-on collision**

- **A GCRTA vehicle sideswiping or broad-siding another vehicle**

- **Physical damage greater than $5,000**

RTA GREATER CLEVELAND
REGIONAL TRANSIT AUTHORITY   01/05/98

Figure B-35. Flow Chart for Post-Accident Testing Process[31]

FTA DRUG & ALCOHOL TESTING PROGRAM

Post-Accident Testing

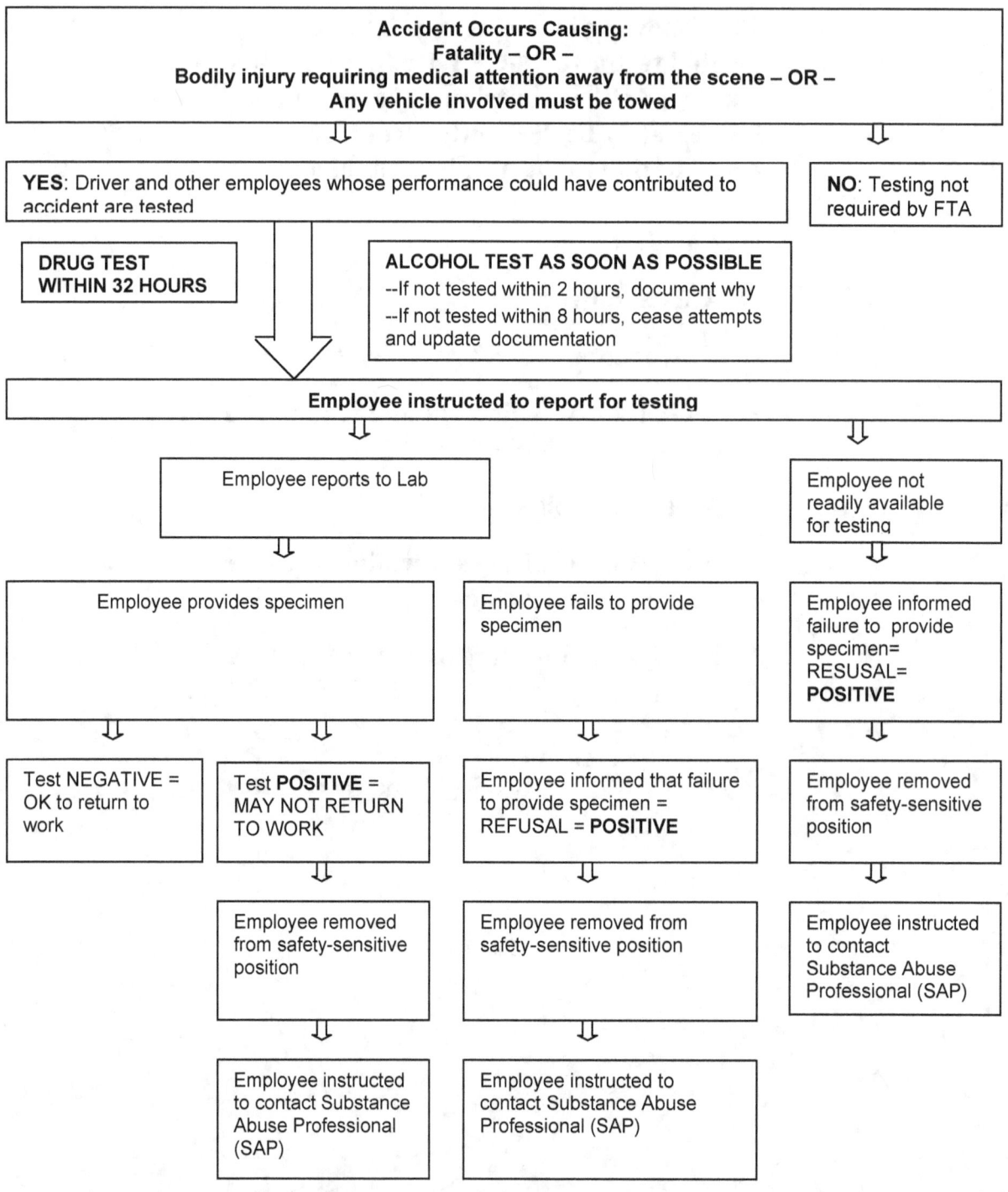

---

[31] West Virginia Department of Transportation (DOT), Division of Public Transit

Figure B-36. Post-Accident Testing Decision Report[32]

POST ACCIDENT TESTING DECISION REPORT

Note: Accident does not necessarily mean collision. If an individual falls on a vehicle and needs to be taken to the hospital, an accident has occurred, and a post-accident test is required unless the driver can be discounted as a contr buting factor. (Spring 1996, *FTA D & A Updates*, p. 5)

System Name: _____

Date of accident: _____   **Time of accident:** _____

Location of accident: _____

Driver of Vehicle: _____**Driver ID No.** _____

WV Uniform Traffic Crash Report Attached   ☐ Yes   ☐ No

1. Was there loss of life as a result of the accident?
☐ Yes   **(Requires Testing – No exceptions)**   ☐ No

2. Did an individual suffer a bodily injury and immediately receive medical treatment away from the scene of the accident?
☐ Yes **(Requires Testing unless question 4 applies.)**   ☐ No (Requires no testing under FTA authority.)

3. Was there disabling damage to any of the vehicles involved? Disabling damage means damage which precludes the departure of any vehicle from leaving the scene of the occurrence in its usual manner in daylight after simple repairs; or damage to any vehicle that could have been operated but which would have further damaged the vehicle if so operated. *Disabling damage does not include damage that could be remedied temporarily at the scene of the occurrence without special tools or parts; tire disablement even if no spare tire is available; or damage to headlights, tail-lights, turn signals, horn, or windshield wipers that makes them inoperative.*
☐ Yes **(Requires Testing unless question 4 applies.)**   ☐ No (Requires no testing under FTA Authority.

4. Can the driver or any other covered employee on the vehicle be completely discounted as a contributing factor to the accident? Note: *If you discount the driver as a contributing factor, it should be well documented.*
☐ Yes   ☐ No   *Even if you answer No, under FTA regulations you must also meet the criteria questions 1, 2, and/or 3 to require testing.*

5. If drug and alcohol testing is required, can the performance of any other safety sensitive employees (e.g., maintenance personnel, dispatcher, etc.), **whose performance may have contributed to the accident** (as determined by the transit agency at the time of the accident), **be completely discounted as contributing to the accident?**
☐ Yes   ☐ No   *Even if you answer No, under FTA regulations you must also meet the criteria questions 1, 2, and/or 3 to require testing. List other employees tested on back of form.*

6. Did you perform a drug and/or alcohol test? ☐ Yes ☐ No **If No, complete #6 and sign and submit a report.**
Name of Supervisor making this determination _____
Time Employee was informed of this determination _____

7. Decision to Test: FTA Authority ☐   **Company Authority** ☐

8. Was an alcohol test performed within 2 hours?   ☐ Yes   Date & Time:_____
☐ No   Why, Not?_____

9. If no alcohol test was performed and more than eight hours elapsed from the time of the accident, please explain._____ _____

10. Was a drug test performed within 32 hours?   ☐ Yes   Date & Time:_____
☐ No   Why, Not?_____

11. Did the driver leave the scene of the accident without just cause?   ☐ Yes   ☐ No
If Yes, please explain _____

Report Submitted By:

_____   _____
                    Signature & Title   Date
For your files, attach test results summary, order to test, chain of custody (USDOT), and alcohol test form (USDOT) WVDPT 11/00

---

[32] West Virginia Department of Transportation (DOT), Division of Public Transit

Figure B-37. Post Accident Testing Procedure[33]

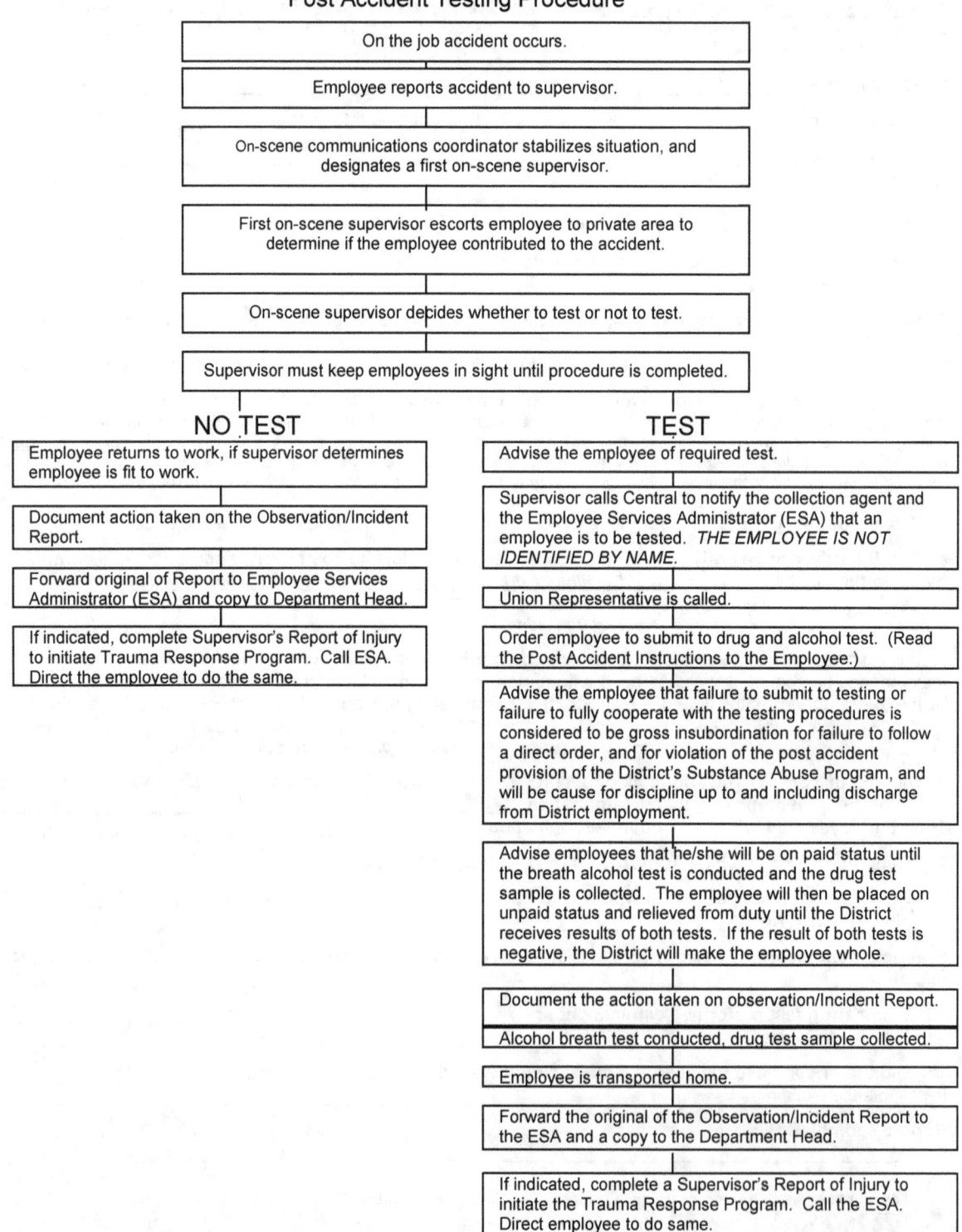

Substance Abuse Program
Post Accident Testing Procedure

On the job accident occurs.

Employee reports accident to supervisor.

On-scene communications coordinator stabilizes situation, and designates a first on-scene supervisor.

First on-scene supervisor escorts employee to private area to determine if the employee contributed to the accident.

On-scene supervisor decides whether to test or not to test.

Supervisor must keep employees in sight until procedure is completed.

NO TEST

Employee returns to work, if supervisor determines employee is fit to work.

Document action taken on the Observation/Incident Report.

Forward original of Report to Employee Services Administrator (ESA) and copy to Department Head.

If indicated, complete Supervisor's Report of Injury to initiate Trauma Response Program. Call ESA. Direct the employee to do the same.

TEST

Advise the employee of required test.

Supervisor calls Central to notify the collection agent and the Employee Services Administrator (ESA) that an employee is to be tested. *THE EMPLOYEE IS NOT IDENTIFIED BY NAME.*

Union Representative is called.

Order employee to submit to drug and alcohol test. (Read the Post Accident Instructions to the Employee.)

Advise the employee that failure to submit to testing or failure to fully cooperate with the testing procedures is considered to be gross insubordination for failure to follow a direct order, and for violation of the post accident provision of the District's Substance Abuse Program, and will be cause for discipline up to and including discharge from District employment.

Advise employees that he/she will be on paid status until the breath alcohol test is conducted and the drug test sample is collected. The employee will then be placed on unpaid status and relieved from duty until the District receives results of both tests. If the result of both tests is negative, the District will make the employee whole.

Document the action taken on observation/Incident Report.

Alcohol breath test conducted, drug test sample collected.

Employee is transported home.

Forward the original of the Observation/Incident Report to the ESA and a copy to the Department Head.

If indicated, complete a Supervisor's Report of Injury to initiate the Trauma Response Program. Call the ESA. Direct employee to do same.

---

[33] San Francisco Bay Area Rapid Transit District (BART)

Figure B-38. Post-Accident Drug and Alcohol Testing Decision Maker Form (Front)

LOS ANGELES COUNTY
METROPOLITAN TRANSPORTATION AUTHORITY

POST-ACCIDENT DRUG AND ALCOHOL TESTING
DECISION MAKER FORM

The MTA *Alcohol & Drug Abuse Policy* (HR 4-2) and the Federal Transit Administration (FTA) regulations (49 CFR Parts 653 and 654) require that employees involved in a vehicle accident (as outlined in the Policy) submit to tests for alcohol and prohibited drugs as soon as possible following the accident. The Policy also requires the testing of any other employee whose performance could have contributed to the accident, as determined by the manager or supervisor at the scene using the best information available at the time of the decision. The testing of non-safety sensitive employees comes under the MTA's own authority.

Accident Information:

Date of Accident_____   Time of Accident: _____

Employee Name: _____ Badge _____ Div/Dept. _____

Decision Questions:

- Was there a fatality? Yes _____ No _____. <u>If *Yes*, Post-Accident tests are required</u>.
- If there was **no** fatality, ask the following questions:

    1. Has any individual suffered a bodily injury and immediately received medical treatment away from the scene of the accident? Yes _____ No _____
    2. If the vehicle involved was a bus, electric bus, van, or automobile, was there a disabling damage as a result of the occurrence and the vehicle was transported away from the scene by a tow truck or other vehicle? Yes _____ No _____
    3. If the vehicle involved was a rail car, trolley car, or trolley bus, was the vehicle removed from revenue service as a result of the accident? Yes_____ No _____

If you checked *Yes* for questions 1, 2 or 3, a Post-Accident test is required unless you determine, using the best information available at the time of the decision, that the employee's performance can be completely discounted as a contributing factor to the accident. (Any reason for NOT conducting a Post-Accident test after you've answered *Yes* to any of the above questions MUST be documented on the reverse side of this form.)

Employee taken to _____ Clinic (nearest medical facility)

by _____ Title_____ at_____ a m./p.m.

FTA regulations also require that alcohol testing must be done as soon as possible following the accident. **If alcohol testing is not conducted within 2 hours after the accident, you must document the reason for the delay on the reverse side of this form. If the alcohol test is not administered within 8 hours, and the drug test within 32 hours, you must cease all efforts to administer the tests and document the reason(s) why the tests were not administered within the FTA-prescribed time frames.**

Figure B-38. Post-Accident Drug and Alcohol Testing Decision Maker Form (Back)

Reason Test Was Not Completed or Delayed:

_____
_____
_____
_____
_____
_____
_____

Testing Procedures:

_____ Determine if employee requires medical attention.

_____ Notify Operations Dispatch that the employee will be sent for 10-58 and briefly state the reason for testing.

_____ Bring employee into a private setting if possible and inform him/her that (s)he will be transported to an MTA-authorized medical clinic for a drug and alcohol test, in accordance with DOT-mandated procedures outlined as Attachment 3 to the *Alcohol & Drug Abuse Policy.*

_____ Complete the *Medical Authorization for Services* form and mark **Post-Accident** for test type.

_____ Escort the employee to the nearest medical clinic and inform him/her that (s)he will be removed from any safety-sensitive function pending the outcome of the tests.

_____ If employee refuses to submit to testing, inform employee that refusal to comply or cooperate is considered an admission of guilt, treated as a positive test, and will result in discipline up to and including termination. Suspend employee pending disciplinary hearing.

Notify Human Resources:

FTA regulations require the Drug & Alcohol Program Manager to keep copies of all documents pertaining to FTA-mandated tests in a centralized location. Upon completion of this form, send the original to Jessica Gil in Human Resources (99-4-4) in a **confidential** envelope and keep a copy in the employee's department/division personnel file.

Please respect the privacy of the employee and the integrity of the testing program. Keep all matters confidential and discuss only with those who "have a need to know."

_____   _____
On-Scene Decision Maker   Title

_____   _____
Date   Department/Division

Figure B-39. Post-Accident Testing Record of Decision (Front)

Southeastern Pennsylvania Transportation Authority								
RECORD OF DECISION **FTA/SEPTA POST-ACCIDENT DRUG AND ALCOHOL TEST**								

DATE OF ACCIDENT:	DAY:	LOCATION:

NAME OF EMPLOYEE:	OCCUPATION:

ACCOUNT NUMBER:	SOCIAL SECURITY NUMBER	INCIDENT NUMBER:
		MM DD YY

VEHICLE NUMBER:	ROUTE:	BLOCK:

TYPE OF VEHICLE:

☐ Bus	☐ Trackless Trolley	☐ Non-Revenue Service Vehicle
☐ LRV	☐ Subway/Elevated	☐ Transit Police Vehicle
☐ N-5	☐ Supervisor T-Car	☐ Other _____

TEST DETERMINATION

Use this table to indicate the results of the accident and the type of test that is required. Check **one** of the boxes that specifies the results of the accident. Do not check more than one box.

	VEHICLE ACCIDENT RESULTS	**TYPE OF TEST**
1.	☐ Revenue vehicle with fatality	FTA POST-ACCIDENT
2.	☐ Revenue vehicle with injury requiring medical treatment away from scene **AND** employee could have contributed	FTA POST-ACCIDENT
3.	☐ Revenue vehicle with any vehicle towed **OR** disabling damage **AND** employee could have contr buted	FTA POST-ACCIDENT
4.	☐ Non-revenue vehicle operated by CDL holder with fatality	FTA POST-ACCIDENT
5.	☐ Non-revenue vehicle operated by CDL holder with injury requiring medical treatment away from scene **AND** employee could have contr buted	FTA POST-ACCIDENT
6.	☐ Non-revenue vehicle operated by CDL holder with any vehicle towed **AND** employee could have contributed	FTA POST-ACCIDENT
7.	☐ Non-revenue vehicle operated by non-CDL holder with fatality	SEPTA POST-ACCIDENT
8.	☐ Non-revenue vehicle operated by non-CDL holder with injury requiring medical treatment away from scene **AND** employee could have contr buted	SEPTA POST-ACCIDENT
9.	☐ Non-revenue vehicle operated by non-CDL holder with disabling damage **AND** employee could have contributed	SEPTA POST-ACCIDENT
10.	☐ Post-accident criteria <u>NOT</u> met. Go to Record of Decision, Reasonable Suspicion Drug and Alcohol Test (Form F0189)	

FINAL DETERMINATION (CHECK [√] ONE FROM ABOVE DETERMINATION.)

☐ FTA Post-Accident Test

☐ SEPTA Post-Accident Test

☐ No Post-Accident Test

Figure B-39. Post-Accident Record of Decision (Back)

RECORD OF DECISION
FTA/SEPTA POST-ACCIDENT DRUG AND ALCOHOL TEST

STATUS OF THIS EMPLOYEE (CHECK [√] ONE.)

☐ Operating the Vehicle
☐ On duty on the Vehicle at the time of the accident
☐ Other Covered Employee

ACCIDENT INFORMATION

ARE ANY OTHER EMPLOYEES TO BE TESTED BECAUSE OF THIS ACCIDENT?

☐ Yes   ☐ No   ☐ Unknown, Investigation indicates possble involvement by others.

Name:	Location:

HOW WAS THIS EMPLOYEE INVOLVED IN THE ACCIDENT?

TIME OF ACCIDENT:	TIME OF TEST (Medical):	ELAPSED TIME (Medical):	
AM PM		AM PM	HR(S) MINS

ALCOHOL TEST GIVEN WITHIN TWO HOURS?:

☐ Yes   ☐ No   If no, state reason below, if known.

SUPERVISOR'S NAME (PRINT):	WORK LOCATION:	ACCOUNT NUMBER:

SUPERVISOR'S SIGNATURE:	WORK EXTENSION:

NOTE: This document must accompany the employee to Medical and be retained on file as a record of decision on whether to administer a post-accident test.

Figure B-40. Post-Accident Documentation Summary Form[34] (Front)

To Be Completed by Supervisor
Return to Department Program Coordinator
within 24 Hours of the Accident.

POST-ACCIDENT
DOCUMENTATION SUMMARY

1) Accident Report #: _____

2) Incident Report #: _____

3) Location of Accident: _____
_____
_____

4) Brief Description: _____
_____
_____

5) Accident Date: _____   Time: _____

6) Report Date: _____   Time: _____

7) Name of Employee: _____

8) Identification Number: _____

9) Position: _____

10) Result of Accident:

    10)a)   Was there a fatality?   ____Yes ____No

    10)b)   Was there disabling damage* to City or other vehicles?   ____Yes ____No

    10)c)   Was anyone transported from the scene for medical attention?   ____Yes ____No
                If yes, what category? ____ Employees
                                        ____ Passengers
                                        ____ Other Vehicle
                                        ____ Other

11) Was the employee sent for a post-accident drug and alcohol test?   ____Yes ____No

12) If no, explain: _____
_____
_____

13) Decision to Test:
    13)a) DOT Authority (transit revenue service or commercial motor vehicles)   ____Yes____No
    13)b) Company Authority (other City equipment, machines, or vehicles)   ____Yes____No

Disabling damage means damage which precludes departure of any vehicle from the scene of the occurrence in its usual manner in daylight after simple repairs. Disabling damage includes damage to vehicles that could have been operated but would have been further damaged if so operated, but does not include damage which can be remedied temporarily at the scene of the occurrence without special tools or parts, tire disablement without other damage even if no spare tire is available, or damage to headlights, taillights, turn signals, horn, mirrors or windshield wipers that makes them inoperative.

---

[34] City of Albuquerque

Figure B-40. Post-Accident Documentation Summary Form (Back)

14) Type of Test: _____ Drug _____ Alcohol

15) Supervisor Making Determination: _____

16) Notification of Test: Date: _____   Time:_____

17) Drug Test Conducted: Date: _____   Time:_____

18) Alcohol Test Conducted: Date: _____   Time_____

19) Did the employee refuse the test? _____Yes _____No
   If yes, please explain: _____
   _____
   _____

20) Did the alcohol test occur more than two hours from the time of the accident? _____ Yes _____No
   If Yes, Explain:_____
   _____

21) If no alcohol test occurred because more than eight hours elapsed from the time of the accident, please
   explain:_____
   _____

22) Did the employee leave the scene of the accident without just cause? _____ Yes _____ No
   If Yes, explain: _____
   _____
   _____

23) If no drug test was performed because more than 32 hours had passed since the time of the accident,
   explain why:
   _____
   _____
   _____

To Be Completed By SAPM

24) Test Result: _____ Positive   _____ Negative   _____Test Cancelled

25) Attachments:
   # Test Result Summary
   # Order to Test
   # Chain of Custody
   # Alcohol Testing Form
   # Return Form to Supervisor Within 24 Hours of Accident

   _____
   Supervisor's Signature

Figure B-41. Failure To Administer Post-Accident Drug Test[35]

> **PREPARE THIS FORM ONLY WHEN THE EMPLOYEE IS NOT TESTED WITHIN 32 HOURS OF THE DETERMINATION THAT A POST-ACCIDENT DRUG TEST IS REQUIRED.**

Names of _____ (insert name of transit system, state, contractor or sub-recipient) safety-sensitive employees involved in the accident/incident:

_____

_____

_____

(first names, middle initials, last names).

Date of accident/incident satisfying at least one of the FTA thresholds requiring post-accident drug testing: _____ (month, day, year)

Time of qualifying accident/incident: _____ AM PM (circle one)

Specific location of the qualifying accident/incident: _____

_____

_____

_____

Reason why the drug test was not administered (check all that apply):

❑ Safety-sensitive employee refused to be tested.
❑ Safety-sensitive employee was medically incapacitated.
❑ Safety-sensitive employee was arrested.
❑ Safety-sensitive employee was detained by law enforcement official.
❑ Other: _____

Specific disciplinary action (if any) taken by _____ (insert name of transit system, state, contractor or sub-recipient):

_____

_____

_____

_____

Date on which this report is completed: _____ (month, day, year).

Name of company official completing and filing report:
_____ (first name, middle initial, last name).

Title of company official completing and filing report:

_____

---

[35] Sioux Falls [South Dakota] Transit System (SuTran).

Figure B-42. Post-Accident Test Master Log [36]

POST-ACCIDENT TEST MASTER LOG

Accident Number	Employees Involved	Position*	Accident Result**	Notify SAPM (F-9)	Test Authority*****	Accident Time	Accident Date	Notification Time	Notification Date	Drug Test Time	Drug Test Date	Drug Test Result (F-4)***	Alcohol Test Time	Alcohol Test Date	Alcohol Test Result (BATI)****	Reason If No Test

* Position   O - Operator; D - Dispatcher; M - Maintenance; S - Security; C - CDL Holder; F - Fire; P - Police; R - Correction

[36] City of Albuquerque

RANDOM TESTING

Figure B-43. Flow Chart for Random Testing Process [37]

FTA DRUG & ALCOHOL TESTING PROGRAM

RANDOM TESTING

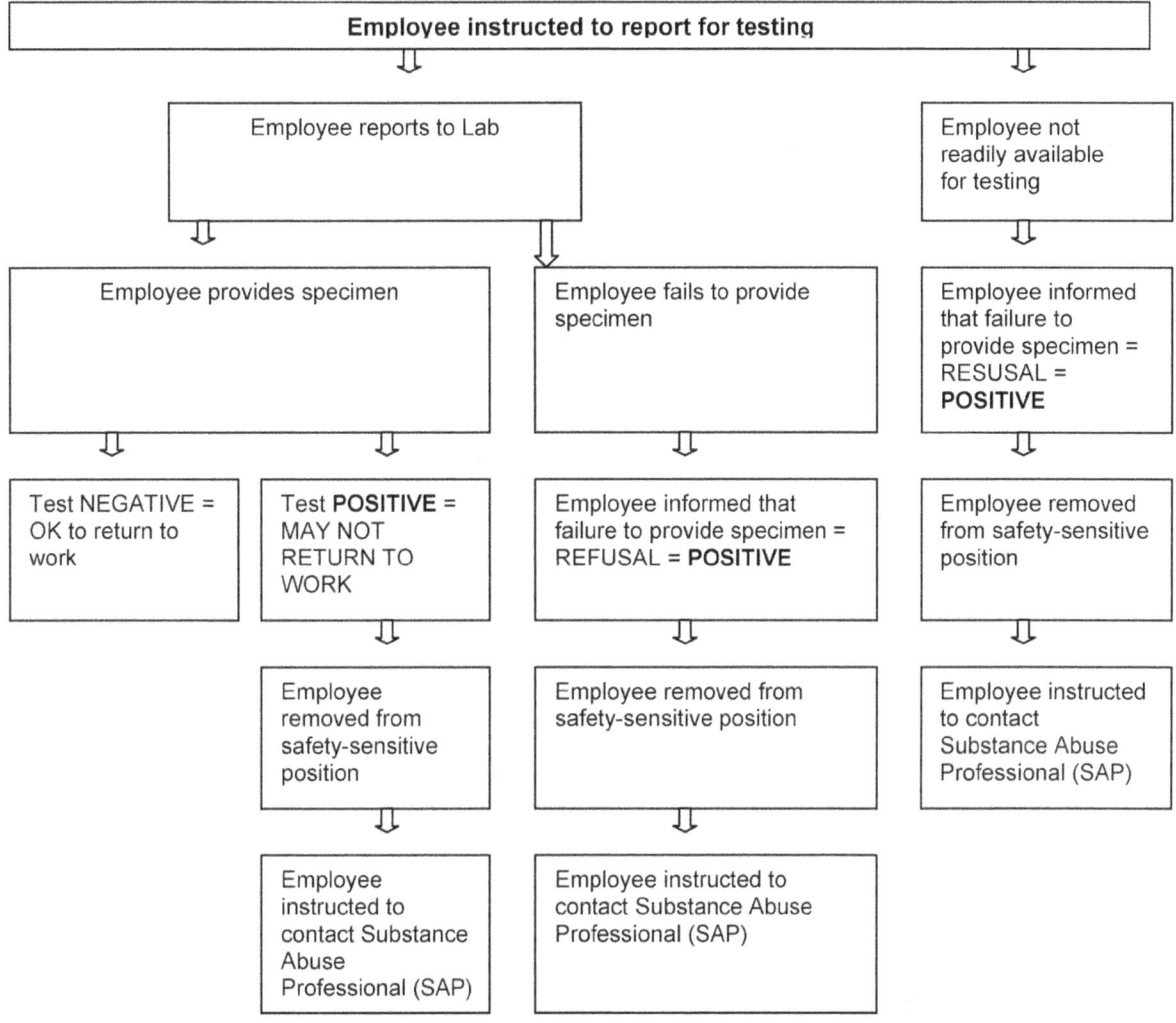

---

[37] West Virginia Department of Transportation (DOT), Division of Public Transit

Figure B-44. Random Testing Procedure[38]

Substance Abuse Program
Random Testing Procedure

Supervisor notified of employee selection for testing.

Notify the employee of selection for random testing, and have the employee stop work.

Order the employee to submit to drug and alcohol tests. (Read the Random Selection Instructions to Employee.)

Advise the employee that failure to submit to or cooperate with drug or alcohol tests, and to sign a consent to test or a release of information form is considered gross insubordination and violation of the random testing provision of the District's Substance Abuse Program, and will be cause for discipline up to and including discharge from District employment.

Inform the employee of availability of rehabilitation at the employee's expense, no need to admit with first positive random test, must admit to drug or alcohol use prior to the second positive test.

Inform the employee that a positive drug or alcohol (0.04% or greater) or refused test will result in disciplinary action up to and including discharge for gross insubordination and violation of the random testing provision of the District's Substance Abuse Program, if the employee has not elected the rehabilitation option prior to the second random positive test.

Escort employee to collection area, and wait for the collection agent to arrive.

Document any unusual activity relating to the drug or alcohol test on the Observation/Incident Report. Forward the original to the Employee Services Administrator (ESA), and a copy to the Department Head.

The supervisor remains with employee and collector until the collection is completed.

NEGATIVE ALCOHOL TEST
The employee returns to work.

LEVEL 1 – ALCOHOL TEST 0.02% TO 0.039%
Advise the employee he/she is relieved of duty for at least eight (8) hours without pay.

LEVEL 2 – POSITIVE ALCOHOL TEST ABOVE 0.04%
Advise the employee he/she is relieved of duty or is on unpaid leave. Transport the employee home. Direct the employee to call ESA for an appointment. The employee will not be allowed to return to duty until released by ESA.

---

[38] San Francisco Bay Area Rapid Transit (BART) District

Figure B-45. Random Drug/Alcohol Testing Notification Form[39]

RANDOM DRUG / ALCOHOL TESTING NOTIFICATION FORM

Employee Identification	
Employee Name:	
Employee ID No.	Social Security No.:
Department	Location:

Selection, Notification, and Testing	
Date Test Scheduled: / /	Test Scheduled: ALCOHOL / DRUG
Supervisor:	Time Employee Notified: am / pm
Date Supervisor Notified: / /	Date Tested: / /
Time Supervisor Notified: am / pm	Time Tested: am / pm

You have been selected for random testing for the presence of prohibited drugs and/or to participate in a breath alcohol test in accordance with Federal regulations for the random drug and alcohol testing of safety sensitive employees. Under District policy, the first time you test positive on a random drug or alcohol (0.04% or greater) test, you may elect rehabilitation at your own expense if you are eligible. It is not necessary for you to admit to drug or alcohol use prior to the test. However, with a second random positive test, you must admit to drug use and/or alcohol abuse prior to the test in order to be eligible for rehabilitation. Even if you admit to drug use and/or alcohol abuse, you may elect rehabilitation at your own expense only if you are eligible. If you do not admit to drug and/or alcohol use prior to the test and either test is positive, it will be cause for disciplinary action, up to and including discharge from District employment.

You will remain in paid status until after the breath alcohol test is conducted and the drug test sample is collected. If the alcohol breath test is negative, you will be released to return to duty. If the breath test reveals a confirmed result between 0.02% and 0.039%, you will be relieved from duty on non-pay status for 8 hours or until your next shift. If the breath alcohol test is confirmed positive (0.04% or greater), you will be relieved from duty, placed in non-pay status, and directed to the Employee Services division of the Human Resources Department for evaluation. If your test result(s) indicate drug use or alcohol abuse, you may be required to participate in a substance abuse rehabilitation treatment program as a condition of continued employment.

Refusing to provide a specimen, tampering with your specimen, or providing false information on a specimen collection or breath alcohol chain of custody form constitutes insubordination and is grounds for disciplinary action, up to and including termination from employment.

_____	_____
Employee Signature	Date/Time
_____	_____
Witness Signature	Date/Time

Original – Employee Services
Yellow - Employee
Pink - Collector

---

[39] San Francisco Bay Area Rapid Transit (BART) District

Figure B- 46. Employee Notice for Random Substance Abuse Test

Massachusetts Bay Transportation Authority
EMPLOYEE NOTICE FOR SCHEDULED SUBSTANCE ABUSE TEST

DATE:

FROM: MBTA Random Drug & Alcohol Program
                Drug and Alcohol Program Administrator

TO:

AT:

TEST DATE: _____(Random Drug Test)

Urine Collection Location:

Appointment Time: _____
Authority for Test: __ DOT/FTA Regulations   ___MBTA Regulations

==

Your name has been selected for a urinalysis drug testing by a computerized program of random selection. Your selection does not imply that this company has a specific cause to suspect you of using illegal drugs. Nonetheless, the DOT Anti-Drug regulations and this company's Anti-Drug Program require that the random testing urine specimen be collected.

You may provide the 60 ml (2 oz) urine specimen in the privacy of a stall. If you are unable to provide a specimen of sufficient quantity, you will be given a waiting period and encouraged to drink water. If you are unable to provide the specimen within the waiting period, you will be deemed to have refused to provide the specimen.

If you refuse to provide the specimen, adulterate the sample, substitute the urine of another person, or fail the drug test, you will be relieved of your employment duties and referred to this company's Employee Assistance Program. You may also be subject to disciplinary action, possibly including termination.

This copy will be retained in your confidential drug testing files, together with the Medical Review Officer's final determination of the drug test results.

Please sign the bottom of this notice to acknowledge its receipt.

Please list any/all medications here.

_____

_____

NOTIFICATION RECEIVED _____   _____
                             Employee Signature   Date and Time

Figure B-47. Random Selection Instructions[40]

Random Selections

1. **Risk Management – Random Selector -** Maintains random pools – (FTA, FHWA, other). When put in payroll system Department Program Coordinator (DPC) indicates who is "safety-sensitive" by job code.

2. Biweekly (consistent with payroll period), the **Random Selector** will determine the number of tests to be drawn from each pool. The numbers will be drawn and reported on form **R-1** for each DPC. The report will also include the type of tests to be conducted.

3. The DPC will research the work schedule of each employee drawn and schedule the tests over the biweekly testing period. The DPC will be careful to distribute the tests throughout the day, day of the week, and testing period. The DPC will keep the list confidential and will not provide any advance notice to the employee. On the day before the test the DPC will notify the appropriate Division Contact to schedule the test using form **R-2**. If the employee is not working on that day, the DPC and division contact will select another time within the testing period. The employee will not be notified of the test until he/she is instructed to immediately proceed to the collection site.

4. The Division Contact person will ensure that the employee is tested at the scheduled date and time. The Division Contact will complete form **R-2** and return it the DPC.

5. The DPC will record on **R-1** the date and time the test was scheduled, if the test was completed or cancelled, and the explanation if no test was performed. The DPC will keep a copy of **R-1** and send the original to the Random Selector within one week of the period end.

6. The Random Selector notes the number of completed tests and will adjust the number of tests to be conducted during the next testing period to account for any missed tests.

7. The DPC will complete a, "Random Individual Test Summary Sheet" (**R-3**), for each random test; will attach appropriate documentation, and will file in the DPC's file.

---

[40] City of Albuquerque

Figure B-48. Roles and Responsibilities of Random Selector[41]

ROLES AND RESPONSIBILITIES
RANDOM SELECTOR

— Maintains random pools for FTA, FHWA, and other City employees

— Coordinates with payroll to ensure pools are accurate and up-to-date, and that all employees are in the right pool

— Determines the number of draws to be performed for each pool reflecting required testing rates adjusted for incomplete tests from prior testing period

— Performs biweekly draws and informs appropriate DPC of numbers selected

— Documents draws and tracks which tests were conducted

— Notifies DPC/SAPM of any procedural violations that compromise the integrity of the random process

Figure B-49. Random Testing Schedule[42]

Transit Department: Random Testing Schedule

Draw Date: _____   Division Contact: _____   Division Notification Date: _____

Draw No.	Employee Name	Scheduled		Employee Notified		Tested		Comments
		Test Date	Test Time	Date	Time	Date	Time	
1.								
2.								
3.								
4.								
5.								
6.								
7.								
8.								
9.								
10.								
11.								
12.								
13.								
14.								
15.								
16.								

---

[41] City of Albuquerque
[42] City of Albuquerque

Figure B-50. Random Testing Selection Documentation Form[43]

Random Testing Number Selection Documentation Form

☐ FTA   ☐ FHWA   ☐ Public Safety   ☐ Other

Department: _____

Test Period Number _____

(A) Number of Safety-Sensitive Functions _____   **(B)** Number of Testing Period Per Year _

(C) Number of Drug Tests this Period ((A) * 50% ÷ (B)) ___   **(D)** Adjusted Number of Tests from Previous Period
Alcohol Tests this Period ((A) * 10% ÷ (B)) ___   _____ Drugs _____ Alcohol

(E) Total Tests (C + D) _____ Drugs _____ Alcohol   Reason for Adjustment: _____

_____

Driver Name or I.D Number	Type of Test D/A/B	Collection Date	Time of Collection	Test Completion *		If No Test Explanation
				Drug	Alcohol	

Total Drug _____   *Y= Yes; N= No; C= Cancelled
Total Alcohol _____

Confidential – For Internal Use Only

---

[43] City of Albuquerque

Figure B-51. Individual Random Test Summary Sheet [44]

RANDOM TESTING
INDIVIDUAL TEST SUMMARY SHEET

Employee Name: _____

Employee Number: _____

Testing Period: _____

Selection Date: _____   Selector: _____

Test Type: _____ Drug   _____ Alcohol

Notification: Date: _____   Time: _____

Test: Date _____   Time: _____

Shift Placement: _____ Begin   _____ Middle   _____ End

**Drug
Test Result:** _____ Negative   _____ Positive   _____ Cancelled

**Alcohol
Test Result:** _____ Below 0.02   _____ 0.02 - 0.039   _____ 0.04 or greater

Consequences: _____ Removal from SS Duty   _____ Referral to SAP   _____ Second Chance   _____ Termination

Attachments:
- ☐ Test Result Summary Form
- ☐ Consent Form
- ☐ Chain of Custody
- ☐ Alcohol Test Form
- ☐ Test Result Documentation
- ☐ SAP Referral Form
- ☐ Other _____

---

[44] City of Albuquerque

Figure B-52. Random Test Master Log [45]

RANDOM TEST
MASTER LOG

Name of Individual Selected	Employee Number	Testing Period	Type of Test Drug	Type of Test Alcohol	Date of Selection	Date of Notification	Time of Notification	Date of Test	Time of Test	Shift Placement	Reason if no Test was Conducted	Results	Comments

---

[45] City of Albuquerque

Figure B- 53. Employee Status Form[46]

This form must be used to add/delete employees to/from the drug and alcohol testing pool for the Rhode Island Public Transit Authority and to change employee information.

Employee Name:

_____

Employee Social Security Number:

_____

Employee Identification Number:

_____

ADD EMPLOYEE TO DRUG AND ALCOHOL TESTING POOL (NOTE THAT A NEGATIVE PRE-EMPLOYMENT DRUG TEST RESULT MUST BE RECEIVED BEFORE A PERSON BEING CONSIDERED FOR A SAFETY-SENSITIVE ROLE CAN BE PLACED ON THE PAYROLL AND INCLUDED IN THE DRUG AND ALCOHOL TESTING POOL):

Date Employee Added to Payroll (Hire Date):

_____

Date Employee Added to Pool of Safety-Sensitive Employees:

_____

Date of Birth: _____ (month, day, year)
Home Telephone Number:

_____

Safety-Sensitive Job/Position Title:

_____

DELETE EMPLOYEE FROM DRUG AND ALCOHOL TESTING POOL:

Date Employee Removed from Payroll (Termination Date):

_____

Date Employee Removed from Pool of Safety-Sensitive Employees:

_____

Date of Birth: _____ (month, day, year)
Home Telephone Number:

_____

Safety-Sensitive Job/Position Title:

_____

CHANGE CURRENT EMPLOYEE INFORMATION:

_____
_____
_____
_____

---

[46] Rhode Island Public Transit Authority (RIPTA)

Appendix C. Example Oversight Forms and Lists

This appendix contains best practice examples of forms and lists that have been used successfully to assist with oversight of service agents, contractors, and subrecipients. Each of these examples is referenced and described in Section 4.2. The examples appear in the following figures, by group:

Service Agent Oversight

C-1. Third-Party Administrator Monitoring Form

C-2. Consortium Monitoring Form

Contractor/Subrecipient Oversight

C-3. Contractor Compliance Guidelines

C-4. Contractor Monitoring Form

C-5. Contractor Monitoring Checklist

SERVICE AGENT OVERSIGHT

Figure C-1. Third-Party Administrator Monitoring Form[1] (Sheet 1)

**FTA Drug and Alcohol Third Party Contractor Checklist
for Compliance with FTA Requirements**

Transit System: _____

Name of Person Completing Form: _____

Review Date: _____

Contractor: _____

Address: _____

_____

_____

Substance Abuse Program Manager: _____

Telephone Number: _____

Management Training

		<u>YES</u>	<u>NO</u>
1.	Have all pertinent safety-sensitive supervisors received the required reasonable suspicion training, 60 minutes for signs and symptoms of alcohol abuse and 60 minutes for signs and symptoms of drug abuse?	☐	☐
2.	Are training certificates in Drug and Alcohol Program files? Information should include type of training, date of training, location of training, and name of instructor.	☐	☐
3	Does contractor have procedures in place to train all new hires and transfers into supervisory positions prior to the time they actually perform duties where reasonable suspicion determinations might be required?	☐	☐

Safety-Sensitive Employee Training

4.	Have all FTA covered safety-sensitive employees received at least 60 minutes of training on the effects of drug use and the indicators of drug use?	☐	☐
5.	Are training certificates in Drug and Alcohol Program files? Information should include type of training, date of training, location of training, and name of instructor.	☐	☐
6.	Are there procedures in place to ensure that all new hires or transfers receive the training as soon as possible after hire date of transfer (i.e., at employee orientation?)	☐	☐

---

[1] Minnesota Department of Transportation

Figure C-1. Third-Party Administrator Monitoring Form (Sheet 2)

Policy

		YES	NO
7.	If policy was not standard Mn/DOT developed policy, was company policy presented to Office of Transit for review and approval?	☐	☐
8.	Which contractor representative/staff reviewed the policy (include titles)?		

_____

_____

_____

_____

9.	Has policy been signed and dated by contractor governing board/owner?	☐	☐
10.	Are previous signed and dated policies on file?	☐	☐
11.	Has policy been distributed to all safety-sensitive employees covered by FTA requirements?	☐	☐

Services

Collection Site:

Name _____

Address _____

_____

Phone number _____

DHHS certified Lab:

Name _____

Address _____

_____

Phone number _____

Medical Review Officer (MRO)

Name _____

Address _____

_____

Phone number _____

Does contractor have a file copy of the MRO's license and other qualifications? ☐ ☐

Figure C-1. Third-Party Administrator Monitoring Form (Sheet 3)

Substance Abuse Professional (SAP)

Name _____

Address _____

_____

Phone number _____

	YES	NO
Does contractor have a file copy of the SAP's license and other qualifications?	☐	☐
12. Are blind sample tests performed? If so, how are they performed?	☐	☐

_____

_____

_____

	YES	NO
13. Are collection site facilities inspected?	☐	☐

14. Date of last inspection: _____

	YES	NO
15. Are canceled tests monitored?	☐	☐

16. Number of canceled tests: _____

Reasons for canceled tests: _____

_____

_____

17. What corrective measures have been taken to minimize the number of canceled tests?

_____

_____

_____

Random Selection Process

Describe the random selection process.

_____

_____

_____

_____

_____

18. Who selects the numbers: _____

_____

19. How often are selections made? Circle one (daily, weekly, monthly, quarterly)

Figure C-1. Third-Party Administrator Monitoring Form (Sheet 4)

20. How soon after selections are made are the tests performed? _____
_____
_____

21. Who notifies the employee of the test requirement? _____

22. During what part of the employees' shifts are tests conducted?
Beginning?_____ Middle?_____ End?_____ Combination?_____

23. What type of employee identification is being used for random testing?
_____
_____
_____

24. Number of safety-sensitive employees _____

25. Required number of tests needed to be performed to meet the regulatory requirement for both drug testing (50%) _____ and alcohol testing (10%) _____

Consortium Participants

26. If contractor is part of a consortium, provide the following information.

Consortium name _____

Address _____
_____

Contact person_____

Telephone number_____

Record Keeping

27. Where are the drug and alcohol testing records stored? _____
_____
_____
_____

28. Who has access to these records? _____
_____
_____

	YES	NO
29. Do files contain all required FTA information?	☐	☐

Figure C-2. Consortium Monitoring Form[2] (Sheet 1)

"Sample"

Drug and Alcohol Consortium Monitoring for Compliance with FTA Requirements

Transit Agency: _____

Name of Person Completing Form: _____

Review Date: _____

Consortium

Name of Consortium: _____

Address of Consortium: _____

_____

_____

Contact Person: _____   Telephone: ___( )_____

Date Contract Signed with Consortium: _____

Contract Timeframe: _____

Is signed contract in Transit Agency's files? _____

Procedures and description of how the consortium complies with blind sample requirements:

_____
_____
_____
_____
_____
_____
_____
_____
_____

Procedures consortium uses to monitor canceled tests: _____

_____
_____
_____
_____
_____
_____
_____
_____
_____
_____

[2] Minnesota Department of Transportation

Figure C-2. Consortium Monitoring Form (Sheet 2)

Procedure consortium uses to ensure scientifically valid random-number selection method to select safety-sensitive employees to be tested: _____

_____

_____

_____

_____

_____

_____

_____

Are the test dates spread evenly throughout the year and the draw period in a pattern that is not predictable, including weekend and holiday testing if a safety function is performed?

_____

_____

_____

_____

_____

_____

_____

_____

Is testing evenly distributed throughout the day (i.e., early morning, afternoon, late evening) and shift times (i.e., beginning, middle, end)? _____

_____

_____

_____

_____

_____

_____

_____

Collection Site(s)
Identify all collection sites and days and hours of operation
(attach additional pages if needed)

Name of Collection Site(s): _____

_____

Address: Address of Collection Site(s): _____

_____

Days and Hours of Collection Site Operation: _____

_____

Name of Collection Site(s): _____

_____

Address: Address of Collection Site(s): _____

_____

Days and Hours of Collection Site Operation: _____

Figure C-2. Consortium Monitoring Form (Sheet 3)

DHHS Certified Laboratory –Name of Primary and Back-up DHHS certified Laboratories

Name of Primary Laboratory:_____

Address: _____

_____

Contact Person: _____   Telephone Number: (___)_____

Name of Back-up Laboratory: _____

Address: _____

_____

Contact Person: _____   Telephone Number: (___)_____

Medical Review Officer (MRO)

Name of MRO(s):_____

Business Address of MRO(s): _____

_____

Business Telephone Number: (___) _____

Credentials of MRO verified and on file (Yes/No)_____

Substance Abuse Professional (SAP)

Name of SAP(s):_____

Business Address of SAP(s): _____

_____

Business Telephone Number: (___) _____

Credentials of SAP verified and on file (Yes/No) _____

Evidential Breath Testing (EBT) Device

Name and Model of EBT:_____

Location of EBT: _____

_____

Documentation that EBT has been calibrated: _____

Breath Alcohol Technician (BAT)

Names of Certified BATs: _____

_____

_____

Credentials of BATs verified and on file (Yes/No) _____

CONTRACTOR/SUBRECIPIENT OVERSIGHT

Figure C-3. Contractor Compliance Guidelines (Sheet 1)

LOS ANGELES COUNTY METROPOLITAN TRANSPORTATION AUTHORITY

FEDERAL DRUG AND ALCOHOL TESTING REGULATIONS

CONTRACTOR COMPLIANCE GUIDELINES

All contract service providers that perform safety-sensitive functions (as defined by Federal Transit Administration {FTA} rules) for the MTA must comply with the FTA drug and alcohol testing regulations (49 CFR Part 655) and the U.S. Department of Transportation (DOT) Procedures for Transportation Workplace Drug and Alcohol Testing Programs (49 CFR Part 40). **Non-compliance shall result in suspension or termination of contract and/or non-payment of outstanding invoices.**

For purposes of this compliance program, **safety sensitive employees** are defined as follows:

Those employees whose job functions are, or whose job descriptions include the performance of functions, related to the safe operation of mass transportation service.

The following are categories of safety-sensitive functions:

1. *operating a revenue service vehicle, including when not in revenue service;*
2. *operating a non-revenue service vehicle when required to be operated by a holder of a Commercial Driver's License (CDL);*
3. *controlling dispatch or movement of a revenue service vehicle or equipment used in revenue service;*
4. *maintaining (including repairs, overhaul, and rebuilding) revenue service vehicles or equipment used in revenue service; and*
5. *carrying a firearm for security purposes.*

Any supervisor who performs or whose job description includes the performance of any function listed above is also considered a safety-sensitive employee.

IMPLEMENTATION GUIDELINES

1. The Materiel Department shall ensure that all bids or Requests for Proposals (RFPs) for services that include the performance of safety-sensitive functions as defined above shall include a provision requiring compliance with mandated DOT/FTA drug and alcohol testing regulations. The MTA reserves the right to audit the proposer's drug and alcohol testing program prior to awarding the contract.

2. Prior to start of work, the successful bidder must certify to the Chairperson of the Source Selection Committee (SSC) that his/her firm is in compliance with the DOT/FTA regulations. (Compliance can be achieved through an in-house program or through a consortium.) The certification shall remain in effect during the term of the contract. A copy of the signed certification shall be sent by the SSC Chair to the Drug and Alcohol Program Manager in Human Resources.

Figure C-3. Contractor Compliance Guidelines (Sheet 2)

3. Using the *EZ* format prescribed by the FTA for the annual report (see Appendix B to 49 CFR Part 653 and Part 654), each covered contractor shall send a quarterly drug and alcohol testing report to the Project Manager, with a copy to the Drug and Alcohol Program Manager in Human Resources. The quarterly report must be submitted no later than the 15th of the month following the close of each quarter. Continued payment of contractor invoices by the MTA is contingent upon contractor submission of the required reports on a timely basis and compliance with FTA-mandated rules.

4. On an annual basis, and no later than February 15 of each year, each covered contractor shall submit to the MTA Human Resources Department annual drug and alcohol testing data using the appropriate FTA prescribed forms. The report shall cover testing conducted during the previous calendar year. It shall be addressed as follows:

> MTA Human Resources Department
> One Gateway Plaza
> Los Angeles, CA 90012-293
> Attn: Drug and Alcohol Program Manager

5. The Human Resources Department shall be responsible for filing the contractors' annual reports with the FTA, along with MTA's own testing data. The reports shall be submitted to the FTA no later than March 15 of each year.

6. The Project Manager for each covered contract shall be responsible for the ongoing monitoring of contractor compliance with DOT/FTA regulations, including ensuring that the quarterly and annual reports as described above are submitted on time.

7. On an annual basis, designated staff from the Management Audit Services and Human Resources departments shall audit contractor compliance, which may include site visits, and report their findings to the Executive Officer, Procurement; Deputy Executive Officer, Human Resources; and the Project Manager responsible for the contract and his/her Department Head.

8. The Project Manager shall be responsible for coordinating contractor responses to the audit findings and ensuring that corrective actions are taken on a timely basis.

_____   _____
Office of the CEO   Executive Officer, Human Resources

Revised: 04/23/99

Figure C-4. Contractor Monitoring Form

GREATER CLEVELAND REGIONAL TRANSIT AUTHORITY
Contractor Monitors

Contractor:_____

Month:_____   Date:_____

GCRTA Representative_____Contract Representative_____

Identified Monitor	Met	Incomplete
Monthly Report with dates of tests performed, type of testing performed and results		
Quarterly Collection Site Review		
Quarterly Laboratory QA records on file		
The following items will be reviewed by the contract representative. Signature above verifies compliance with FTA regulations. Quarterly on-site Records Review • Each drug screen has correct Chain of custody • Collection times are monitored to determine that employee goes to the collection site immediately after notification • The collection site performed the correct test using the correct forms. All discrepancies have documentation of the problem and resolution. • Random Selection is spread out throughout the selection period and there is no pattern • All documentation is on file for each Reasonable Suspicion test • Documentation is available for all Post Accident Decisions • Documentation is available for all MRO notifications • The MRO process is in written procedure and is currently used.		
Quarterly review of collection site certification		
Annual certification check of SAP		
Annual certification check of MRO		
Annual certification check of Laboratory		
Annual review of Policy & Procedure		
Annual review of Collection site Policy & Procedure		
Annual review of MRO Policy & Procedure		
Annual review of SAP Policy & Procedure		

Figure C- 5. Contractor Monitoring Checklist[3] (Sheet 1)

FTA Drug and Alcohol Contractor Checklist

Contractor: _____

Substance Abuse Program Manager: _____

Address: _____

_____

Telephone Number: _____

Management Training

1. Did a representative of your company attend any management training on how to set up a substance abuse testing program? If so, please provide the following information:

Type of Training	Date of Training	Location of Training	Name of Instructor

Policy

2. Was your company policy presented to the FTA Grantee for review and approval?

3. Which Company representative/staff reviewed the policy (include titles)?

_____

_____

4. Did legal counsel review your policy?   Yes _____   No _____

5. Please attach a copy of your recent policy.

6. Has your Governing Board approved your **revised policy**?   Yes _____   No _____
    If yes, when _____
    Please attach a copy of your Governing Board approval.

Reasonable Suspicion Training

7. Did any of your transit supervisors attend a qualified Reasonable Suspicion Training Program:
    Yes _____   No _____
    (60 minutes of the signs and symptoms of drugs and 60 minutes on the signs and symptoms of alcohol)

If yes, please list attendees below.

_____

[3] Ohio Department of Transportation

Figure C-5. Contractor Monitoring Checklist (Sheet 2)

Employee	Length of Training	Date & Location of Training	Name of Instructor

Employee Training

Please provide the following information on the substance abuse awareness training program to your employees. (Please attach agenda)

Employee	Length of Training	Date & Location of Training	Name of Instructor

8.   Have you had new hires since employee training was conducted?   Yes _____   No _____

9.   Did you provide the new hires with substance abuse awareness training?
     Yes _____   No _____   If yes, please provide the following information for each new hire.

Employee	Length of Training	Date & Location of Training	Name of Instructor

If no, when will the training be conducted? _____

10. Please describe the method of instruction and content of new hires' substance abuse awareness training.

Collection Site:

Name _____

Address _____

_____

Phone number_____

DHHS certified Lab:

Name _____

Address _____

_____

Phone number_____
(Please attach copy of DHHS certificate)

Figure C-5. Contractor Monitoring Checklist (Sheet 3)

Medical Review Officer (MRO)

Name _____

Address _____

_____

Phone number _____
(please attach resume and a copy of license and other qualifications)

Substance Abuse Professional (SAP)

Name _____

Address _____

_____

Phone number _____
(please attach resume and a copy of license and other qualifications)

11. How are blind sample tests performed?

12. Do you inspect your collection site facilities?   Yes _____   No _____

13. Date of last inspection: _____

14. Do you monitor canceled tests?   Yes _____   No _____

15. Number of canceled tests _____

16. Reasons for canceled tests: _____

_____

_____

_____

17. What corrective measures have been taken to minimize the number of canceled tests?

_____

_____

_____

Equipment

18. Is alcohol testing contracted out?   Yes _____   No _____
    If yes, please provide the following information on the vendor/agency.

Name _____

Address _____

_____

Phone number _____

Figure C-5. Contractor Monitoring Checklist (Sheet 4)

Type of device used (specify Make and Model #) _____

19. Are non-evidential testing devices being used?   Yes _____   No _____

20. Describe the procedures used for conducting alcohol testing: _____
_____
_____
_____

21. Type and location of primary EBT: _____

22. Type and location of backup EBT: _____

23. Provide list of certified Breath Alcohol Technicians (BAT) or Screen Test Technicians (STT):

Name	Date of Certification	Date of Last Training

24. Please attach a copy of the BAT/STT training certificate.

Random Selection Process

Please describe the random selection process.
_____
_____
_____
_____
_____

25. Who selects numbers?

26. How often are selections made (daily?, weekly?, Monthly?, Quarterly?)

27. How soon after selections are made are the tests performed?

28. Who notifies employee of test requirement? During what part of the employees'
    Shift are tests conducted? Beginning? _____   Middle? _____   Combination? _____

29. What type of employee identification is being used for random testing? _____
_____

30. Number of safety-sensitive employees _____

31. Required number of tests needed to be performed to meet the regulatory requirement for both drug testing
    (50%) _____ and alcohol testing (10%) _____

Figure C- 5. Contractor Monitoring Checklist (Sheet 5)

32. Please list all agencies or departments that are included in your random testing pool. For each agency indicate the name, title, and phone number of the person who oversees it:

Agency/Department	Contact Person	Title	Phone #

Turnkey Participants

33. If you hired a contractor to provide all or part of the testing services for you, please identify the service provider:

Company_____

Contact Name _____

Address _____

_____

Phone Number _____

34. Please describe the procedures for monitoring turnkey contractor:_____
_____
_____

Consortium Participants

35. If you are part of a consortium. Please provide the following information.

Consortium Program Manager _____

Address_____
_____Phone Number _____

36. Please provide a description of the consortium (who is involved, who oversees, etc.)
_____
_____
_____

Consortium Participants

37. If you are part of a consortium, please provide the following information.

Consortium Program Manager _____

Address_____
_____ Phone Number _____

Figure C-5. Contractor Monitoring Checklist (Sheet 6)

38. Please describe the consortium (who is involved, who oversees, etc.)

_____

_____

_____

39. Please describe the distribution of responsibilities within the consortium (who is responsible for what).

_____

_____

_____

Record Keeping

40. Where are the drug and alcohol testing records stored? _____

_____

_____

_____

41. Who has access to these records? _____

_____

_____

_____

42. Do you maintain the following records?
    a. Data on test results that have a BAC of 0.02 or greater
    b. Employer's copy of the alcohol test form
    c. Data on test refusals
    d. Documents presented by a covered employee to dispute the result of an alcohol test
    e. Data on referrals to SAP
    f. Record pertaining to determination by a SAP concerning a covered employee's need for assistance
    g. Records concerning a covered employee's compliance with the recommendations of the SAP
    h. Calibration documentation for evidential breath testing device
    i. Annual MIS report
    j. Records pertaining to evaluations
    k. Data regarding training of employees
    l. Data regarding training of BATs
    m. Collection process (including logbooks, if used)
    n. Data on test results that are less than 0.02

Reporting

43. Please indicate the dates the annual MIS reports were sent to the grantor.

Certification of Compliance

44. Please attach your certification of compliance.

Appendix D. Example Specimen Collection Forms and Lists

This appendix contains best practice examples of forms and lists that have been used successfully to assist with management of urine and breath collection operations. Each of these examples is referenced and described in Section 4.3. The examples appear in the following figures:

D-1. Employee Instructions for Collection Process

D-2. Drug Test Collection Form

D-3. Shy Bladder Form

D-4. Shy Lung Form

D-5. Collection Site Checklist

Figure D-1. Employee Instructions for Collection Process[1]

Employee Instructions for Collection Process

PLEASE TAKE A FEW MINUTES TO READ THE FOLLOWING INFORMATION THAT DESCRIBES YOUR ROLE IN THE COLLECTION PROCESS

1. Present a required Photo I.D. to the Collector. If you do not have a Photo I.D., an employer representative will be asked to identify you.

2. Remove any unnecessary garments (coats, jackets, hats, etc.). All purses and briefcases must remain with outer garments.

3. Empty your pockets, and show the contents to the Collector.

4. You will be provided a sealed specimen bottle, and the Collector will unwrap it in your presence.

5. You should observe the entire collection procedure. The Collector will check the specimen for its volume, temperature, and color. The Collector will then seal the bottle.

6. Make sure you have initialed the seal on the specimen bottle.

7. You should complete the information on the Custody form as instructed by the Collector. You will be given a copy after completion.

8. The results of the laboratory analysis will be forwarded to the Medical Review Officer (MRO). If the lab results are negative, the MRO will notify your employer. If the lab results are positive, the MRO will contact you at the phone number(s) you provided, to give you the opportunity to discuss the test results and to submit information concerning the authorized use of the drug(s) in question.

THANK YOU. YOUR COOPERATION IS GREATLY APPRECIATED.

---

[1] Ohio Department of Transportation

Figure D-2. Drug Test Collection Form

SAN FRANCISCO BAY AREA RAPID TRANSIT DISTRICT
NIDA DRUG TEST COLLECTION CHECKLIST

COLLECTOR   DONOR

___   1.   Donor identify verified by photo I.D. or employer representative   ___

___   2.   Procedure explained to donor.   ___

___   3.   Donor removed coat, hat, etc. left outside collection area and emptied pockets, but retained wallet.   ___

___   4.   Donor washed hands prior to collection, in view of collector.   ___

___   5.   Collector placed bluing in toilet bowl and tank, and secured all water sources and possible adulterants from donor access.   ___

___   6.   Collection kit was opened in front of donor.   ___

___   7.   Donor was asked to furnish urine specimen. Collector waited outside restroom/stall door until donor exited. Donor was told not to flush toilet.   ___

___   8.   Specimen remained in full sight of BOTH collector and donor until completely packaged. If the specimen was transferred from one container to another, transfer was done in THE PRESENCE AND FULL VIEW OF THE DONOR.   ___

___   9.   In the presence of the donor, the collector checked the specimen for color, sign of contamination, temperature, and quantity. All of the above were conducted within 4 minutes of collection and documented on the chain of custody form.   ___

___   10.   Collector placed lid on container, and tightened it securely IN THE PRESENCE AND FULL VIEW OF THE DONOR.   ___

___   11.   Container was sealed with tamper evident tape in the donor's presence and full view. Donor initialed tape. Collector verified the information on the label as identical to the chain of custody form attached to the specimen bottles. DONOR MUST SIGN NAME THE SAME WAY EACH TIME.   ___

___   12.   Chain of custody form was signed by donor, and donor was given a copy.   ___

___   13.   Donor was allowed to wash hands.   ___

Donor and collector agree that all of the above procedures have been completed, and the urine submitted is that of the donor signed below and has not been tampered with.

_____ _____   _____ _____
Collector Signature   Date   Donor Signature   Date

_____   _____
Print Collector Name   Print Donor Name

Figure D-3. Shy Bladder Form[2]

SHY BLADDER CHECK LIST

DOT 3 Hour Time Limit Check List

Donor's Name: _____

Collector's Initials:_____

1. _____ The start time should be indicated on the COC. This starts with your first attempt. (Example: donor arrives at 12:00; he/she has until 3:00 to void.)

2. _____ The donor can have up to 40 ounces of fluids. The actual total mount must be recorded under the remarks section, as well as the time of each attempt to void.

3. _____ If the donor cannot void in three hours, call the company representative and explain to them that the DOT regulations require the donor have a physical examination to determine if there is a physical reason for this.

4. _____ Can the evaluation be performed at the testing facility? If so, schedule the evaluation as soon as possible.

5. _____ If the inability to void is not a result of a physical or pre-existing psychological disorder, the test will be considered a test refusal. If there is a medical condition, the test is cancelled unless it is a pre-employment test. The doctor should determine if the medical problem is a result of a long-term or permanent disability. If a disability is found, the MRO should conduct an exam to identify any signs of illegal drug use (a blood test is permitted). If no illegal drug use is found, the test should be designated as negative.

If no Doctor is available:

1. _____ Make an appointment for the evaluation at a later date, but as soon as possible.

2. _____ Ask the employer what their procedure is.

---

[2] Ohio Department of Transportation

Figure D-4. Shy Lung Form[3]

SHY LUNG CHECKLIST

You need to try and get the donor to complete testing before getting this far. You may even want to let another BAT try and speak with and instruct the donor. Sometimes, another person's view can help.

Donor's Name: _____

Collector's Initials:_____

1. _____Call the company contact and explain the situation. Just as in a drug screen situation, the donor must be examined to determine if there is a medical problem. Can the evaluation be performed at the testing facility?

2. _____If it can be performed at the collection site, schedule the examination as soon as possible.

3. _____If Doctor finds a medical problem, the test will be cancelled and the company informed. The Doctor must provide written documentation to the company explaining the reason.

If no Doctor is available:

1. _____Make an appointment for the evaluation at a later date, but as soon as possible.

2. _____Ask the employer what their procedure is.

---

[3] Ohio Department of Transportation

Figure D-5. Collection Site Checklist[4] (Sheet 1)

COLLECTION SITE CHECKLIST

System Name _____

Collection Site _____

Date _____

Drug Testing Procedures

SPECIMEN COLLECTION

Does the collection site(s) meet the Department of Transportation requirements published in 49 CFR Part 40, *Procedures for Transportation Workplace Drug and Alcohol Testing Programs*?

Does the collection site check the donor's ID? Does the collection site have a procedure in place to confirm donor identity when no ID is presented (i.e., supervisor attests to identity)?

Does the collection site:

— Provide a privacy enclosure for urination, a void receptacle, a suitable clean writing surface, and a water source for hand washing, which, if practicable, should be outside the privacy enclosure?;

— Secure the privacy enclosure when not in use or, if this is not possible (e.g., when a public restroom is used), visually inspect it prior to specimen collection to ensure that unauthorized persons are not present and that there are no unobserved entrance points?;

— Have restricted access during specimen collection?;

— Add a bluing agent to the toilet water to prevent dilution of the specimen;

— Secure the toilet tank top or blue tank water;

— Turn off, tape, or prevent the use of other sources of water (e.g., sink or shower) that are located in the privacy enclosure where urination occurs?;

— Remove all potential adulterants; and

— Secure areas suitable for concealing contaminants such as trash receptacles, paper towel holders, etc.?

Does the collection site have a procedure in place for notifying the employer if the employee does not report for the test in the designated time frame?

Do you have a procedure to notify the collection site of the identity and contact information of the Designated Employer Representative (DER)?

Does the collection site use the correct USDOT Chain of Custody and Control forms for DOT/FTA tests (and only DOT tests)?

---

[4] Ohio Department of Transportation

Figure D-5. Collection Site Checklist (Sheet 2)

Is the specimen and CCF under the control of the collector throughout the collection process? Is the collector the only person that handles the specimen before it is sealed?

Are "limited access" signs posted in areas of public access?

Does the collection site restrict access to specimens and specimen collection materials?

Are collection sites available to perform collections during all days and hours that the transit system performs safety-sensitive job duties?

Do collectors recheck the privacy enclosure following the collection process?

Split Sample

Is the split specimen procedure being utilized at the collection site? After the specimen has been collected, it must be divided into two specimen bottles (30 ml of urine in one primary specimen bottle and 15 ml in the split specimen bottle) in the presence of the donor. If the primary test returns a positive test result, the employee can request that the split sample be tested at a separate DHHS laboratory.

Are procedures in place to have a split sample transferred to a second HHS lab for analysis? Have you established a business relationship with the second HHS lab to ensure that split specimens will be processed in a timely manner and that the employer will provide payment for the split analysis (subject to reimbursement by the employee)?

Insufficient Volume of Specimen

Is the collection site following the correct procedures if the employee being tested is unable to produce a sufficient amount of urine for the test?

- — Discard the original specimen.
- — Obtain another urine sample within three hours of the previous test. The employee cannot drink more than 40 ounces of fluid during the three hours.

Does the employer direct the employee to have a medical examination within 5 days if 45 ml cannot be provided within three hours?

Does the medical physician provide the MRO with a statement indicating whether or not the insufficient specimen was the result of a genuine medical condition?

Does the MRO notify the employer in writing of the medical examination conclusion?

If there is no medical explanation for the insufficient specimen, is the test regarded as a refusal to be tested?

Figure D-5. Collection Site Checklist (Sheet 3)

For a pre-employment test that results in insufficient volume, is a contingent offer of employment made prior to the medical evaluation?

For a pre-employment insufficient volume test, does the medical evaluation determine if the shy bladder was due to a long-term or permanent disability? Does the medical examination look for signs of illegal drug use? If no signs of illegal drug use are found, does the MRO verify the test as negative?

Observed Collections

Are procedures in place to require the collection site personnel to conduct a mandatory observed collection immediately after the first collection in the following circumstances?

- The employee's urine sample is outside the normal temperature range;
- The collection site person observes conduct that clearly and unequivocally indicates an attempt to adulterate or substitute the sample;
- Following a positive, adulterated, or substituted test, the split sample is not available for testing; or
- The specimen is invalid with no medical explanation.

Does the transit system, at its option, have a procedure to determine if an observed collection will be conducted in the following circumstances?

- The employee has previously been determined to have used a controlled substance without medical authorization and the particular test is being conducted under the FTA regulation as a return to duty or follow-up test.

Does the collection site have both genders available in case an observed collection is necessary?

Is the employee told the reason for an observed collection if one is performed?

Privacy/Confidentiality

Does the collection site have adequate measures in place to protect the privacy of the employee and the integrity of the collection process?

Does the collection site and Medical Review Officer have adequate measures in place to communicate confidential matters to designated individuals at the employer?

Appendix E. Example Medical Review Forms and Lists

This appendix contains best practice examples of forms and lists that have been used successfully to assist with management of the medical review process. Each of these examples is referenced and described in Section 4.4. The examples appear in the following figures:

E-1. Roles and Responsibilities of Medical Review Officer

E-2. MRO Checklist

E-3. MRO/Donor Interview Checklist

E-4. Request To Test Split Sample

E-5. Failure To Make Contact Notification

E-6. MRO Verification Flow Chart

Figure E-1. Roles and Responsibilities of Medical Review Officer [1]

ROLES AND RESPONSIBILITIES
MEDICAL REVIEW OFFICER

— Detailed knowledge of testing procedures defined in 40 CFR Part 40, as amended.

— Detailed knowledge of laboratory analysis procedures and report interpretation

— Receive test results from the laboratory and verify lab report and assessments-
  - Specimen identification
  - Certifications (donor, collector, certifying scientist)
  - Chain-of-custody complete
  - Administration items complete

— Review and interpret each confirmed positive test result.

— Notify donor of positive test result and provide an opportunity for donor to discuss positive test results, and discuss as needed.

— Review donor's medical history and medical records as appropriate.

— Notify DPC and SAPM of verified positive test.

— Process donor's request for analysis of the split specimen.

— When applicable, provide input to SAP on return-to-duty decision.

— Conduct medical assessment on applicants with insufficient volume due to a long-term or permanent disability.

— Conduct physical examinations for evidence of illegal drug use on employee with an opiate positive test when analytical results are inconclusive.

— Administratively review each negative test result.

— Order re-tests as appropriate when the accuracy or validity of a positive test result is questionable.

— As appropriate, order a full adulteration panel including specific gravity, creatinine concentration, and PH when the integrity of the specimen is in question (i.e., temperature out of range, collector observes questionable behavior).

Request laboratory to conduct confirmatory analysis for methamphetamine to distinguish use with the active ingredient in over-the-counter medications.

---

[1] City of Albuquerque

Figure E- 2. MRO Checklist[2] (Sheet 1)

Donor's Name:_____ ID#:_____

Specimen ID#:_____ Date of Collection:_____

Positive Result Reported: Date_____   Time_____

A. REVIEW DOCUMENTS

☐ Yes   ☐ No   1. Are the Chain-of-Custody (COC) forms filled out correctly?

☐ Yes   ☐ No   2. Does the information that appears on the lab COC form match the information on the MRO form?
- Compare the specimen identification number contained on the both the laboratory copy and the MRO copy of the COC.
- Compare the employee ID # and SS# on both forms to insure they are the same.

If No,   ☐ Request the laboratory records regarding the specimen to determine if the correct laboratory procedures were followed; or
☐ Require the retest of the specimen

Lab Contact: _____

Phone #: _____

Date: _____

Comment: _____

If the specimen identification number or employee ID# is not the same, the result should not be reported at this time. Do not verify the positives until you are fully satisfied that the results reported are those for the specimen identified to the subject donor. If unsure, order a retest and have the certifying scientist personally inspect the original specimen container to ensure it was properly accessioned.

☐ Yes   ☐ No   3. Did the collector complete the required certification of the COC?

☐ Yes   ☐ No   4. Did the donor complete the require certification on the COC?

☐ Yes   ☐ No   5. Did the certifying scientist complete the required certification on the COC?

☐ Yes   ☐ No   6. If the donor did not sign the COC, did the collector properly note the declination and record the explanation (if any)?

☐ Yes   ☐ No   7. Is the COC block completely and legibly completed?

☐ Yes   ☐ No   8. Is all other information completed properly?

B. VERIFY LABORATORY RESULT AND ASSESSMENT

☐ Yes   ☐ No   9. If methamphetamine positive, request isomer concentrations (d = Rx, l = otc).

☐ Yes   ☐ No   10. If opiate positive, request codeine and morphine concentrations.

If over 2000 ng/ml, order 6-MAM.

Lab Contact Person: _____

Phone #: _____

Date: _____

Comment: _____

☐ Yes   ☐ No   11. As necessary request: _____ Concentration Data

_____ Validity Tests   _____ Adulteration Panel

_____ Other, Specify: _____

---

[2] City of Albuquerque

Figure E-2. MRO Checklist (Sheet 2)

C. DONOR CONTACT

☐ Yes ☐ No 12. Document attempts to contact donor.

	Date	Time	Phone #	Contact	Comment	Initials
1.						
2.						
3.						
4.						
5.						

☐ Yes ☐ No 13. If unable to contact donor, contact employer representative.

Employer Contact: _____ Date _____ Time _____

☐ Yes ☐ No 14. If more than 72 hours have passed since the employee was notified by employer or 10 days have passed from the date the result was reported, verify the result as positive.

D. EMPLOYEE INTERVIEW

☐ Yes ☐ No 15. Hello, my name is Dr. Christenson, the Medical Review Officer for the City of Albuquerque.

☐ Yes ☐ No 16. Verify Employee Identity

_____ Am I talking to _____? (employee name) Yes _____ No _____

_____ Did you have a drug screen on _____ (date) at _____ (location)? Yes _____ No _____

_____ Were you satisfied that the specimen you gave was collected, labeled, and sealed in your presence? Yes _____ No _____

_____ Can you tell me your SS# and birth date? SS#: _____
Birth Date: _____

☐ Yes ☐ No 17. "The reason I am speaking to you personally is because the results of the drug test have been received and it is a positive test. The purpose of this interview is to provide you an opportunity to voluntarily share information with me that might explain a positive result, such as anything from your medical history, prescriptions, recent treatment or something in your diet. Before I ask you any further questions, I want to tell you that any information that you may disclose will be **TREATED CONFIDENTIALLY** and will not be released unless a DOT regulation requires or permits such a disclosure. (Information obtained that indicates you are not fit for duty will be reported to your employer.) You have the option of not discussing the matter with me if you choose. Do you have any questions at this point?"

☐ Yes ☐ No 18. Did the employee refuse to discuss the test result or decline the interview with the MRO? Yes _____ No _____

If yes, verify the test as positive and explain: _____

_____

_____

☐ Yes ☐ No 19. "I need to ask you some questions about your medical history to determine whether or not your drug test results could have been caused by medication you may have been taking."

Figure E-2. MRO Checklist (Sheet 3)

Prescription Drugs:

	Rx	Rx	Rx	Rx
Rx #				
Date				
Doctor				
Quantity				
Drug				
Pharmacy				
Phone				
Rx Phone				

Over-the-Counter Drugs:

Drug Name			
Quantity			
Usage			
Comment			

Diet:

Product			
Quantity			
Usage			
Comment			

Dental, ENT, Opthalmolopic, Other Procedure:

Procedure		
Date		
Doctor		
Comment		
Phone		

☐ Yes ☐ No   20. Inquire about illicit drug usage: _____

_____

☐ Yes ☐ No   21. Request for Medical Records when appropriate: _____

_____

☐ Yes ☐ No   22. Request an exam on in-person interview when appropriate -
Appointment Date: _____
Appointment Time: _____
Physician: _____

☐ Yes ☐ No   23. If there is no legitimate medical explanation, tell the donor your conclusion:
Notification Date: _____   Time: _____

Figure E-2. MRO Checklist (Sheet 4)

☐ Yes   ☐ No   24. Notify the donor that they may request analysis of the split specimen at their expense. The request must be made within 72 hours.

☐ Yes   ☐ No   25. Did you tell the donor the procedure for requesting the split analysis (i.e., telephone numbers, contact person)?   Yes _____   No _____

☐ Yes   ☐ No   26. Notify the donor that if requested, the split specimen will be sent to Another certified laboratory and tested for presence of the same drug(s). The cost of the test is $_____ *

Split Analysis   _____   Declined   Laboratory _____
_____   Requested   Date Requested _____
_____   Specimen ID#   Result _____

*Note: If the donor requests the split analysis, but indicates they cannot afford to pay, proceed with the test.

☐ Yes   ☐ No   26. Inform the donor of consequences of a positive test and where to obtain a list of resources for resolving problems associated with alcohol or drugs and where to receive a referral for an assessment by a substance abuse professional.

☐ Yes   ☐ No   27. Offer to answer any questions; give name and phone number.

☐ Yes   ☐ No   28. Notify donor of split analysis and of verified test result.

Date: _____   Time: _____   Result: _____

E. MRO VERIFICATION

Employee Name: _____   SS#: _____
City/Department: _____   Dept. Contact: _____
Date of Interview: _____   Contact Phone #: _____
Verification completed & employee notified of results: Date _____ Time _____
Employee Notified of Results: Date _____   Time _____
Employer Contact If Other Than Above: _____
Test Result Report Form Sent to Employee Contact: _____
Results Reported As: _____ Positive, Drug _____
_____ Negative, (Scientifically Insufficient)
_____ Negative
_____ Cancelled, Specify _____
Comments:

_____
MRO's Signature: _____
MRO Name: _____
MRO Date: _____

☐ Complete Chain-of-Custody Form

Figure E-3. MRO/Donor Interview Checklist[3]

MRO/Donor INTERVIEW CHECKLIST

_____ 1. Identify yourself as a physician serving as the Medical Review Officer (MRO) for the City of Albuquerque with the duty of receiving and reviewing drug test results. Clearly state that you have been designated the MRO for the City of Albuquerque drug testing program.

_____ 2. Establish identity of the donor (i.e., full name, social security number of donor I.D. number, date of birth.)

_____ 3. Inform donor that medical information discussed during the interview is confidential, and may only be disclosed under very special circumstances.

_____ 4. If the donor holds a medical certificate under a DOT agency rule, advise the donor that information regarding test results and information supplied by the donor will be provided to the DOT Agency as required by appropriate regulations.

_____ 5. Tell the donor are calling about the specific drug test he/she underwent on the specific date and at the specific location. Inform the donor what drug(s) the specimen tested positive for.

_____ 6. Briefly explain the testing process, discussing screening and confirmation testing, and laboratory reporting.

_____ 7. If the donor request the quantitative levels of the confirmed results, provide them if available. If the quantitative levels are unavailable, the MRO should request them. However, this does not delay his/her verifications decision pending receipt of the quantitative data.

_____ 8. Ask for recent medical history, when appropriate.
_____ Prescription drugs
_____ OTC Drugs
_____ Dental, ENT, Ophthalmologic, or other medical procedures.
_____ Food Ingestion

_____ 9. Request donors provide medical records or documentation of prescription for controlled substance when appropriate. Set a specific deadline for receipt of the medical records.

_____ 10. Request donors undergo a medical examination or evaluation, when appropriate. Make arrangements for medical evaluation.

_____ 11. Notify the donor that he/she may request the split specimen be tested, and Explain this process to him/her. Provide information about payment for the split specimen test in accordance with employer's policy, if appropriate. Tell the donor that the split specimen test will not delay reporting of the initial test result to their employer.

_____ 12. If the verification process is complete, inform the donor that they are to report to their Department Program Coordinator.

_____ 13. If the test result was verified positive, inform the donor that they are to report to their Department Program Coordinator.

_____ 14. Offer to answer any further questions.

_____ 15. Give your name and phone number in case the donor has any further questions.

USE THE MRO VERIFICATION WORKSHEET TO DOCUMENT INTERVIEW

---

[3] City of Albuquerque

Figure E-4. Request To Test Split Sample[4]

Split Sample   Date_____

Medical Review Officer

Request to Retest Form
_____

Medical Review Officer: _____

Agency Name: _____

Address: _____

Telephone: _____

Manager's Name: _____

Employee Name: _____

Employee SS #: _____

Employee Address:_____

Employee Telephone No: (Work)_____   (Home)_____

Date of original test: _____

I request that the split specimen of my urine sample provided on _____
be tested for the presence of the following drugs: marijuana, cocaine, opiates, phencyclidine (PCP), and
amphetamines consistent with the requirements specified in 49 CFR Part 40.

The split specimen will be packaged and sent to the following DHHS laboratory for analysis:
(note: This is a different lab than the one which performed the analysis on the primary lab.)

_____

_____

_____

I understand that I may be responsible for all costs of collection, storage, shipment, and examination relating to this
retest.

_____

Employee's Signature

_____

Agency Drug Program Coordinator's Signature

_____

[4] Ohio Department of Transportation.

Figure E-5. Failure To Make Contact Notification [5]

DATE FAXED TO COMPANY   _____
COMPANY NAME: _____
ATTENTION: _____
PHONE NUMBER: _____
DONOR NAME: _____
SSN / EMPLOYEE NUMBER   _____

The above listed employee must speak to an MRO and we have failed to make contact. Therefore, we need your assistance. Please have the donor contact _____ (name of MRO) at _____ (telephone number of the MRO) as soon as possible. It is important that the employee knows the name of the correct doctor for whom to ask.

In accordance with Federal Regulations, we are not permitted to start the "72-hour clock" until we know the donor has been successfully notified. However, in the event the MRO and the employer have been unsuccessful in contacting the donor, the result may be reported as a no contact result after 10 days. In order to start the "72-hour clock", we need to know that you have successfully made contact with the donor advising him/her to contact the MRO. Verbal contact must be made directly with the donor. Messages left with spouses and/or family members do not qualify as notification. Additionally, please note that leaving messages on answering machines, voice mails, pager systems, etc. are likewise not acceptable, as notification.

Please fill in the information below and fax this page to _____ (contact person at MRO's office) at _____ (fax number of contact person) as soon as contact with employee is made.
REMEMBER, THE '72-HOUR CLOCK" MAY NOT START UNTIL WE ARE PROPERLY NOTIFIED THAT THE DONOR HAS BEEN INFORMED TO CONTACT THE MRO.

If you require additional information or have questions pertaining to this correspondence, please call _____ (contact person at MRO's office) at _____ telephone number of contact person).

Please print:

I, _____, (employer/supervisor) hereby attest that _____ (insert name of employee) has been notified to contact the MRO as soon as is possible. I attest that verbal contact was made directly with the donor on _____ (date of contact) and understand that the "72-hour clock" starts from this date.

_____Date_____
(Signature of authorized supervisor or employer)

---

[5] Prepared by University Services, Arsenal Business Center, Building 4, 5301 Tacony St., Philadelphia, PA, 19137, 215 743 4200, for the Monroe County Transportation Authority, East Stroudsburg, PA.

Figure E-6. MRO Verification Flow Chart[6] (Sheet 1)

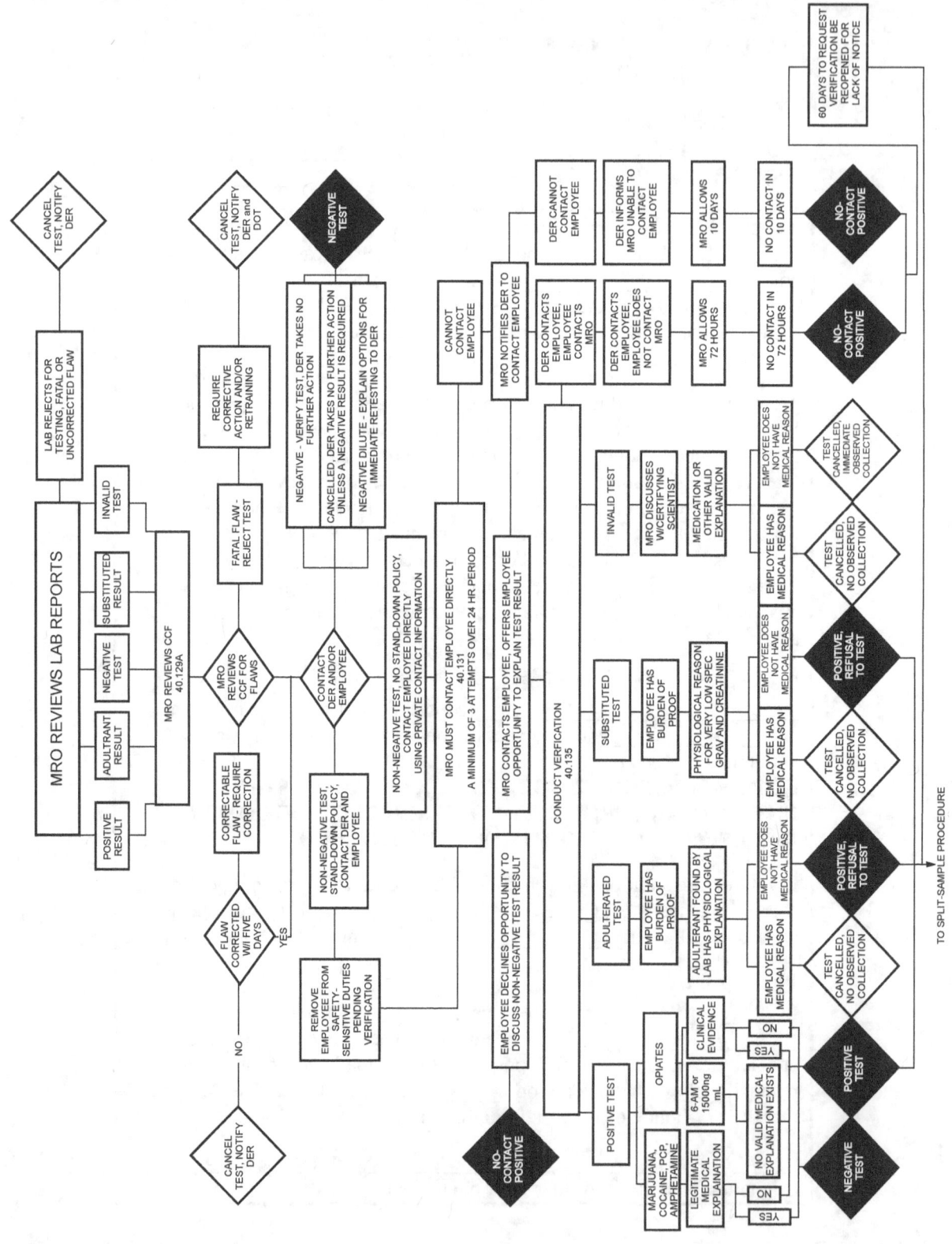

[6] Prepared by the Ketron Division of the Bionetics Corporation

Figure E-6. MRO Verification Flow Chart (Sheet 2)

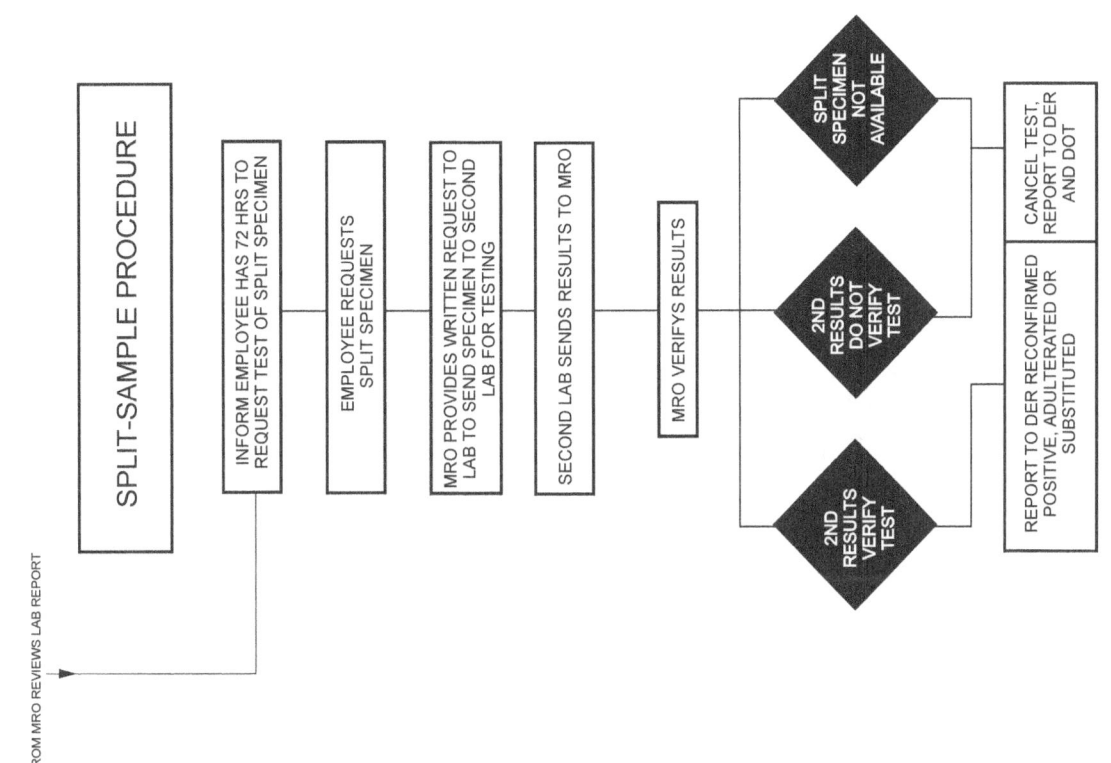

Appendix F. Example Referral, Evaluation, and Treatment Forms

This appendix contains best practice examples of forms that have been used successfully to assist with management of the referral, evaluation, and treatment process for safety-sensitive employees who test positive for drugs or alcohol or otherwise violate provisions of Parts 40 or 655. Each of these examples is referenced and described in Chapter 5. The examples appear in the following figures:

F-1. Referral to Substance Abuse Professional

F-2. Substance Abuse Program Treatment Referral Form

F-3. Agreement for Continuation of Employment

F-4. Return-to-Work Agreement

F-5. Return-to-Duty and Post Rehabilitation Worksheet

F-6. SAP Client Evaluation

F-7. Mandated Individual Treatment Plan

F-8. SAP Return to Work Evaluation

F-9. Follow-Up Assessment

F-10. Return to Duty Testing Flow Chart

F-11. Follow-Up Testing Flow Chart

Figure F-1. Referral to Substance Abuse Professional[1]

SUBSTANCE ABUSE PROFESSIONAL REFERRAL

I acknowledge that I have received a referral to a Substance Abuse Professional as required by FTA regulations.

The cost of this service will be borne by: ☐ the City   ☐ the employee

Substance Abuse Professional referral:

Name_____

Address_____

City/State_____

Phone_____

Alternate Substance Abuse Professional referral:

Name_____

Address_____

City/State_____

Phone_____

I have received a copy of this referral:

_____   _____
Employee Signature   Date

_____   _____
Agency Representative Signature   Date

_____
[1] City of Albuquerque

Figure F-2. Substance Abuse Program Treatment Referral Form

SAN FRANCISCO BAY AREA RAPID TRANSIT DISTRICT
1330 Broadway, Suite 907, Oakland, 94612
(510) 464-6205, (510) 464-6198
Fax # (510) 464-6255

SUBSTANCE ABUSE PROGRAM
TREATMENT REFERRAL FORM

Date_____ Referred To: _____ Phone:_____

Employee Name _____ M/F Birthday _____ Age _____

Address _____ City _____

Zip Code _____ Home Phone _____ Work Phone _____

Job Title: _____Shift _____Days Off _____

Self-Pay: _____ Insurance Carrier: _____ Plan # _____

Group: _____ Phone # _____ Address: _____

BART Pay: _____
(If BART Pay, Submit Claims to Barbara George, BART EAP, 1330 Broadway, Suite 907, Oakland, 94612.)

Circumstances under which employee is being referred: _____

_____

_____

_____

SAP Findings and Recommendations: _____

_____

_____

Please call _____ Phone_____

with findings, recommendations, and name and phone number of the assigned case manager.

Figure F-3. Agreement for Continuation of Employment[2]

POST DRUG and/or ALCOHOL TESTING AGREEMENT
FOR CONTINUATION OF EMPLOYMENT

THIS AGREEMENT is entered into by and between _____(transit system) And _____(employee). _____(transit system) is committed to providing channels of assistance for employees seeking rehabilitation. However, the employee seeking rehabilitation must be committed in his/her efforts to remain free of drug use and alcohol misuse. Therefore, as part of the commitment, it is understood that the employee's continuation of employment at _____ (transit system), for matters relating to the Drug Abuse and Alcohol Misuse Prevention Program, is based upon and constrained by the following terms:

1. _____ (employee) and _____ (transit system) mutually agree that your continuation of employment for the next five years is contingent upon your satisfactorily meeting the terms outlined in this agreement and that failure to do so may subject you to disciplinary action up to and including termination of employment with _____ (transit system).

2. You must submit to evaluation of potential drug and/or alcohol problems by a substance abuse professional (SAP). This evaluation must be completed within _____ days from the date of this document.

3. You must participate in and attend rehabilitation, treatment, or community resource programs recommended by the SAP. The SAP or a program counselor shall provide _____ (transit system) with periodic progress reports regarding your participation and attendance at all required sessions. Failure to follow the terms of the program recommended by the SAP shall be cause for discipline up to and including discharge.

4. Following satisfactory completion of the program recommended by the SAP, you must at a minimum, report to _____ (transit system) within 24 hours following release by your counselor or the SAP and be tested for drug use and/or alcohol misuse before you are allowed to return to duty. Such return to duty test must be negative for drugs and/or show an alcohol concentration of less than .02. There may also be additional stipulations outlined by _____ (transit system) and/or the SAP at this time.

5. During the five (5) year period following your return to duty, you will be subject to unannounced follow-up testing. There will be a minimum of six (6) tests in the twelve (12) months following your return to duty date. Such tests are in addition to any tests necessitated by _____ (transit system) Program or required by the SAP as part of his/her program to monitor your compliance with his/her recommendations.

6. If you are absent from work during the five (5) year period and it is determined that the absence is a result of, or related to, the use of drugs or misuse of alcohol, then _____ (transit system) may take disciplinary measures up to and including discharge.

7. If you violate the conditions of _____ (transit system) Program, the SAP's program, refuse to be tested, or have a positive drug test or an alcohol test with a concentration of .04 or greater under any testing circumstance within the five year period, you will be discharged.

This Agreement is voluntarily entered into by all parties, and in consideration for continuation of employment, the above conditions are hereby agreed to.

Dated this _____ day of _____, 20__.

SIGNATURES:

_____   _____
Employee   **Date**   **Representative**   **Date**

_____

[2] Ohio Department of Transportation

Figure F-4. Return-to-Work Agreement[3]

POST DRUG and/or ALCOHOL TESTING
RETURN-TO-WORK AGREEMENT

THIS AGREEMENT is entered into by and between _____
AND _____. _____ is committed to providing channels of
assistance for employees seeking rehabilitation. However, the employee seeking rehabilitation must be
committed in his/her efforts to remain free of drug use and alcohol misuse. Therefore, as part of the
commitment, it is understood that the employee's continuation of employment at _____,
for matters relating to the Drug Abuse and Alcohol Misuse Prevention Program, is based upon and
constrained by the following terms:

1. _____ and _____ mutually agree that your continuation of
   employment for the next five years is contingent upon your satisfactorily meeting the terms outlined
   in this agreement and that failure to do so may subject you to disciplinary action up to and including
   termination of employment with _____.

2. During this period, you will be subject to unannounced follow-up testing with a minimum of six (6)
   tests the first year. Such tests are in addition to any tests that may be necessitated by
   _____ Drug Abuse and Alcohol Misuse Prevention Program or any tests required by a
   substance abuse professional (SAP) as part of their program to monitor the employee's compliance
   with his/her recommendations. You will be subject to disciplinary action up to and including
   discharge if you refuse to submit to testing or if you test positive for drugs and/or alcohol during this
   time period.

3. If you are absent from work during this period and it is determined that the absence is a result of, or
   related to, the use of drugs or misuse of alcohol, then _____ may take disciplinary
   measures up to and including discharge.

4. If you violate the conditions of _____ Program, the SAP's program, refuse to be
   tested, or have a positive drug test or an alcohol test with a concentration of .04 or greater under any
   testing circumstance within the five year period, you will be discharged.

This Agreement is voluntarily entered into by all parties, and in consideration for continuation of
employment, the above conditions are hereby agreed to.

Dated this _____ day of _____, 20__.

SIGNATURES:

| _____ | | _____ | |
| **Employee** | **Date** | **Representative** | **Date** |

---

[3] Ohio Department of Transportation

Figure F-5. Return to Duty and Post Rehabilitation Worksheet[4]

SAP RETURN TO DUTY AND POST REHABILITATION WORKSHEET

Employee: _____

Employee SSN or ID#: _____

    Address: _____

    Phone (H): _____   Phone (W): _____

Employer Name & Address: _____

_____

Contact Person: _____

    Date of SAP Contact: _____ Date of Assessment: _____

    Date Test Verified: _____

    Type of Test: _____ Random   _____ Reasonable Suspicion

    _____ Post-Accident   _____ Return-To-Duty   _____ Follow-Up

    Substances: _____

Treatment Plan Signed: ☐ Yes ☐ No   Date: _____

Signed Release of Information: ☐ Yes ☐ No   Date: _____

Rehabilitation Program Date Began: _____ Completed _____

Name & Address of Rehab Facility: ☐ Outpatient ☐ Inpatient

Contact Name: _____   Phone: _____

Progress Assessment: _____

_____

☐ Rehab Testing

Date	Results	Date	Results
___	___	___	___
___	___	___	___
___	___	___	___
___	___	___	___
___	___	___	___

Discharge Diagnosis: _____

_____

After Care Plan and Follow-Up: _____

_____

Program Complete or Assessment: _____

_____

☐ Extension of Treatment _____

☐ MRO Input _____

☐ Return-to-Duty Test Date _____ Result _____

☐ Return to Safety-Sensitive Duty Date _____

☐ Return to Duty Contract Date _____

☐ Follow-Up Testing Schedule (Complete on Back) _____

Supervisor _____   Phone _____

Comments _____

---

[4] City of Albuquerque

Figure F-6. SAP Client Evaluation[5] (Sheet 1)

Substance Abuse Professional Client Evaluation

Client: _____

Date: _____

Evaluator: _____

<u>Directions:</u> If one of the following statements says something that is <u>true</u> about you, put a <u>check mark</u> in the space for <u>YES.</u> If a statement says something that is <u>not true</u> about you, put a <u>check mark</u> in the space for <u>NO.</u> Please answer all the questions.

	YES	NO
1. Do you feel you are a normal drinker or drug user?	_____	_____
2. Have you ever awakened in the morning after some drinking or drug use the night before and found you could not remember a part of the evening before?	_____	_____
3. Does your spouse, parents, family (or friends) ever express worry or complain about your drug or alcohol use?	_____	_____
4. Can you stop drinking or using drugs without a struggle?	_____	_____
5. Do you ever feel bad about your alcohol or drug use?	_____	_____
6. Do friends or relatives think you are a normal drinker or drug user?	_____	_____
7. Do you ever try to limit your drinking or drug use to certain times of the day or to certain places?	_____	_____
8. Are you always able to stop drinking or using drugs when you want to?	_____	_____
9. Have you ever attended a self-help meeting of Alcoholics Anonymous (AA) or Narcotics Anonymous (NA)?	_____	_____
10. Have you ever gotten into fights when drinking and/or using drugs?	_____	_____
11. Has drinking or using drugs ever created problems with you and your spouse/partner?	_____	_____
12. Has your spouse (or other family members) ever sought professional help about your alcohol or drug use?	_____	_____

---

[5] Massachusetts Bay Transportation Authority (MBTA)

Figure F-6. SAP Client Evaluation (Sheet 2)

Substance Abuse Professional Evaluation
Page Two
Employee # _____

	YES	NO
13. Have you ever lost friends or partners because of your drug or alcohol use?	_____	_____
14. Have you ever gotten into trouble at work because of your drug or alcohol use?	_____	_____
15. Have you ever lost a job because of your alcohol or drug use?	_____	_____
16. Have you ever neglected your obligations, your family, or your work for two or more days in a row because you were using alcohol or drugs?	_____	_____
17. Do you ever use alcohol or drugs before noon time?	_____	_____
18. Have you ever been told you have medical problems with your liver?	_____	_____
19. Have you ever had withdrawal symptoms, severe shaking, hearing voices, and/or seen things that were not there, after using alcohol or drugs?	_____	_____
20. Have you ever gone to anyone for help about your drug or alcohol use?	_____	_____
21. Have you ever been in a hospital because of your drug or alcohol use?	_____	_____
22. Have you ever been in a psychiatric hospital or on a psychiatric ward in a general hospital where your drug or alcohol use was part of the problem?	_____	_____
23. Have you ever seen a mental health care professional, doctor, social worker or member of the clergy for help in addressing a mental health issue that was or could have been related to your alcohol and/or drug use?	_____	_____
24. Have you ever been arrested due to your alcohol or drug use?	_____	_____
25. Have you ever been arrested for drunk driving?	_____	_____
26. Have you ever experienced financial difficulties because of your alcohol and/or drug use?	_____	_____
27. Do you ever spend more money on drinking or drug use activities than you planned to?	_____	_____
28. Have you ever lied about your drinking or drug use?	_____	_____

Figure F-6. SAP Client Evaluation (Sheet 3)

Scoring Key: Substance Abuse Professional Evaluation

<u>Directions for scoring:</u> Add the point values for all items on which points are earned.

<u>Classification of client:</u> 0-2 (total score), client uses alcohol/drugs in social situations not presenting serious problem, but needs education. 3-5 (total score), client is demonstrating border line use, and should have an educational and treatment intervention referral. 6 and above (total score), client is demonstrating addictive behavior (past or present), and should be assessed for current use and treatment referral.

	YES	NO
1.		2
2.	2	
3.	1	
4.		2
5.	1	
6.		2
7.	2	
8.		2
9.	5*	
10.	1	
11.	2	
12.	2	
13.	2	
14.	2	
15.	2	
16.	2	
17.	1	
18.	2	
19.	5	
20.	5	
21.	5	
22.	2	
23.	2	
24.	2	
25.	2	
26.	2	
27.	2	
28.	2	

*Discretion may be indicated in scoring this item to account for those who accompanied a family member to the meeting.

Figure F-7. Mandated Individual Treatment Plan[6] (Sheet 1)

Date: _____

MANDATED INDIVIDUAL TREATMENT PLAN

He/She has indicated by their Signature below, his/her need to participate in the MBTA Rehabilitation Program. Be advised that participation at ECS does not exempt the employee from performing his/her job responsibilities, nor does adherence to this treatment plan guarantee the employee a Return To Work Agreement or reinstatement to the Authority.

Self Help Group Meetings:

Educational Group Meetings:

Individual Counseling:

Aftercare Program:

Other:

I will participate in the MBTA Rehabilitation Program and agree to Comply with all conditions of my treatment plan.

I understand that an approved Leave of Absence (LOA) for Family Medical Leave Act (FMLA), extended illness, or Worker's Compensation does not preclude my participation in ECS. It is my responsibility to discuss any absences from group or individual treatment due to illness of FMLA with my counselor and the Manager of ECS.

I UNDERSTAND THAT I WILL BE SUBJECT TO PERIODIC DRUG AND ALCOHOL TESTING AT THE AUTHORITY'S DISCRETION.

_____	_____
Employee Signature	Date
_____	_____
Counselor Signature	Date

---

[6] Massachusetts Bay Transportation Authority (MBTA)

Figure F-7. Mandated Individual Treatment Plan (Sheet 2)

RETURN TO WORK SERVICE PLAN

Date _____

Name _____

Employee # _____

Education Group Meetings
List required meetings

_____

_____

_____

EAP Group Meetings
List Required Meetings

_____

_____

_____

Individual Counseling
List Counselor Name or

_____

Referral source. Also list

_____

Frequency of counseling required

_____

After Program (for clients being released from an input. treatment program)

_____

_____

_____

Comments:

_____

_____

_____

_____

_____

_____

_____

_____

_____

Client Initials _____ Counselor Initials _____

Figure F-7. Mandated Individual Treatment Plan (Sheet 3)

INITIAL SERVICE PLAN

_____

Date

_____   _____

Name   **Employee #**

Education Group Meetings
List Required Meetings

_____

_____

_____

EAP Group Meetings
List Required Meetings

_____

_____

_____

Individual Counseling
    List Counselor Name or

    Referral source. Also list

    Frequency of counseling required

_____

_____

_____

_____   _____

EAP REPRESENTATIVE   **Client Signature**

Completed Intake	_____	☐
Completed Assessment Group	_____	☐
Completed Disease Concept Group	_____	☐
Completed Denial Group	_____	☐
Completed Self Help Information	_____	☐
Completed SAP Evaluation (if needed)	_____	☐
Completed MBTA Drug and Alcohol Training	_____	☐

Second Review Scheduled _____   ☐

Reviewed by _____ **Date:** _____

Figure F-7. Mandated Individual Treatment Plan (Sheet 4)

CONTINUING SERVICE PLAN II

Date _____

Name _____   **Employee #**

Education Group Meetings
List Required Meetings
_____

_____

_____

EAP Group Meetings
List Required Meetings
_____

_____

_____

Individual Counseling
   List Counselor Name or
   Referral source. Also list
   Frequency of counseling required
_____

_____

_____

EAP REPRESENTATIVE _____   **Client Signature**

Completed 1ST Review _____   ☐
Completed Job Safety Group   _____   ☐
Completed Stress and Coping Tech. Group   _____   ☐
Completed Family Group   _____   ☐
Completed Road to Recovery   _____   ☐
Third Review Scheduled   _____   ☐

Reviewed by _____   **Date:** _____

Figure F-7. Mandated Individual Treatment Plan (Sheet 5)

CONTINUING SERVICE PLAN III

_____
Date

_____

Name   **Employee #**

Education Group Meetings
List Required Meetings
_____
_____
_____

EAP Group Meetings
List Required Meetings
_____
_____
_____

Individual Counseling
List Counselor Name or
Referral source. Also list   _____
Frequency of counseling required   _____

_____   _____
EAP REPRESENTATIVE   **Client Signature**

Completed 2nd Review   _____   ☐
Completed Relapse Prevention Group   _____   ☐
Completed Aftercare Planning Group   _____   ☐

Transition Meeting Scheduled   _____   ☐

Reviewed by _____ **Date:** _____

Figure F-8. SAP Return to Work Evaluation[7]

Substance Abuse Professional Return to Work Evaluation

Case # _____   Employee Identification # _____

Date of Evaluation: _____

Substance Abuse Professional:_____
                                   Print Name

Describe client's progress with treatment/education plan since being referred for services. What goals were achieved? What areas of concern were addressed? Number of groups attended?

_____
_____
_____
_____
_____
_____

Describe client's attitude and compliance with treatment/educational referral including self-help groups, treatment referrals, and aftercare.

_____
_____
_____
_____
_____

Recommendations for Return to Work aftercare treatment/education and follow-up Drug and/or Alcohol Testing.

_____
_____
_____
_____
_____

# of Drug Tests   1st year ___ 2nd year___ 3rd year___ 4th year ___ 5th year ____

# of Alcohol Tests   1st year ___ 2nd year___ 3rd year___ 4th year ___ 5th year ___

_____   _____
Signature and License #   Date

_____
Mailing Address

_____
Telephone #

_____
[7] Massachusetts Bay Transportation Administration (MBTA)

Figure F-9. Follow-Up Assessment[8]

FOLLOW-UP ASSESSMENT

EMPLOYEE NAME: _____ DATE: _____

WORK LOCATION: _____ SUPERVISOR: _____

REASON FOR INITIAL ASSESSMENT: _____

DATE OF SPECIFIC VIOLATION: _____

DATE OF INITIAL ASSESSMENT: _____

TREATMENT PROVIDER: _____

PRIMARY COUNSELOR _____ PHONE: _____

LEVEL OF CARE: _____

DESCRIPTION OF INITIAL TREATMENT PLAN: _____

_____

INCLUSIVE DATES OF THE TREATMENT PROGRAM: _____

DESCRIBE EMPLOYEE'S LEVEL OF PARTICIPATION IN THE TREATMENT PROGRAM: _____

_____

_____

_____

PROVIDE CLINICAL CHARACTERIZATION OF EMPLOYEE'S INVOLVEMENT WHILE IN TREATMENT:

_____

_____

_____

_____

HAS EMPLOYEE DEVELOPED AN UNDERSTANDING OF THE CONSEQUENCES OF HIS/HER DRUG AND/OR ALCOHOL USE: YES _____ NO _____

HAS THE EMPLOYEE FULLY DEMONSTRATED SUCCESSFUL COMPLIANCE WITH THE INITIAL TREATMENT RECOMMENDATIONS: YES _____ NO _____ IF NO, DESCRIBE: _____

_____

RECOMMENDATIONS FOR FOLLOW-UP TESTING: _____

_____

RECOMMENDATIONS FOR FOLLOW-UP CARE: _____

_____

_____

_____

RETURN TO WORK UA/BAT TEST DATE: _____

RETURN TO WORK AGREEMENT SIGNED: _____

RETURN TO WORK DATE: _____

SUPERVISOR NOTIFIED OF RTW _____ DATE: _____

SAP _____ PHONE: _____

---

[8] San Francisco Bay Area Rapid Transit (BART) District

Figure F-10. Return to Duty Testing Flow Chart[9]

FTA DRUG & ALCOHOL TESTING PROGRAM

<u>Return to Duty Testing</u>

Determination made by Executive Director on advice of Substance Abuse Professional to test under FTA Drug and Alcohol Testing Program

Employee instructed to report for testing

Employee reports to Lab		Employee not readily available for testing
Employee provides specimen	Employee fails to provide specimen	Employee Informed that failure to provide specimen = REFUSAL = **POSITIVE**
Test NEGATIVE = OK to return to work / Test **POSITIVE** = MAY NOT RETURN TO WORK	Employee informed that failure to provide specimen = REFUSAL = **POSITIVE**	Employee removed from safety-sensitive position
Employee removed from safety-sensitive position	Employee removed from safety-sensitive position	Employee instructed to contact Substance Abuse Professional (SAP)
Employee instructed to contact Substance Abuse Professional (SAP)	Employee instructed to contact Substance Abuse Professional (SAP)	

---

[9] West Virginia Department of Transportation, Division of Public Transit

Figure F-11. Follow-Up Testing Flow Chart[10]

FTA DRUG & ALCOHOL TESTING PROGRAM

Follow-up Testing

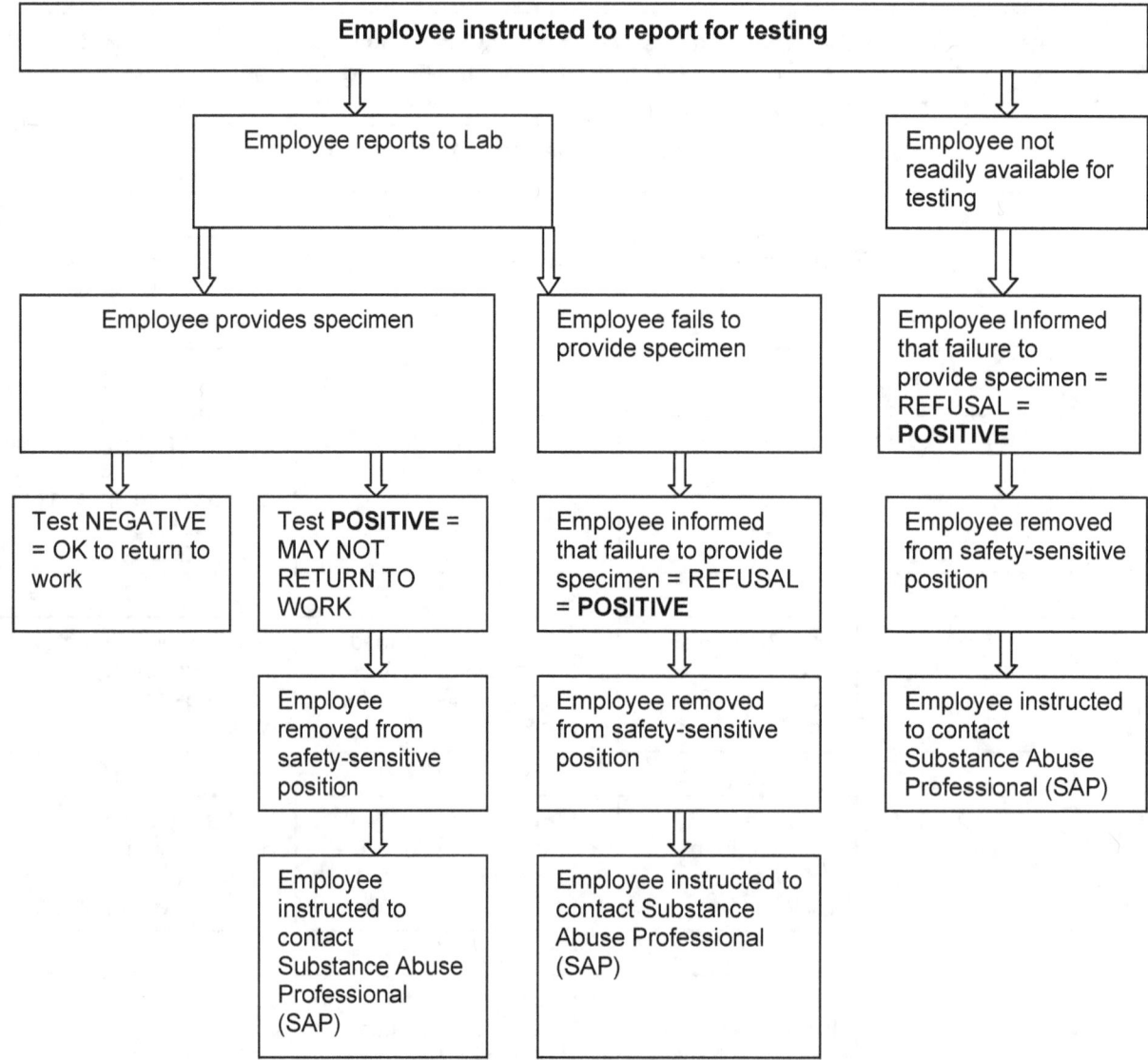

www.ingramcontent.com/pod-product-compliance
Lightning Source LLC
Chambersburg PA
CBHW080407290526
45791CB00008BA/2180